Charles L. Proudfit
February 1982

Psychoanalysis and Old Vienna:

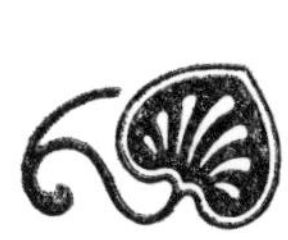

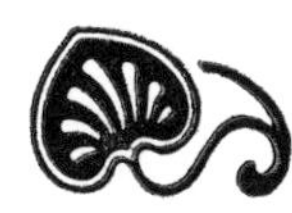

Freud, Reik, Schnitzler, Kraus

SPECIAL ISSUE OF THE PSYCHOANALYTIC REVIEW

Murray H. Sherman
Editor

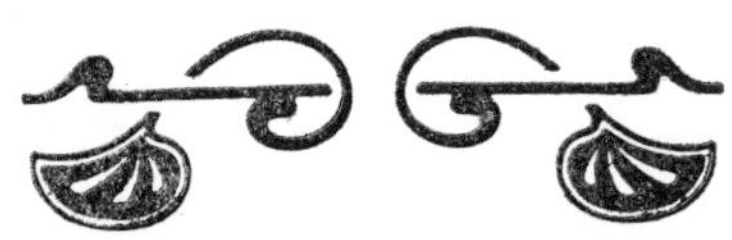

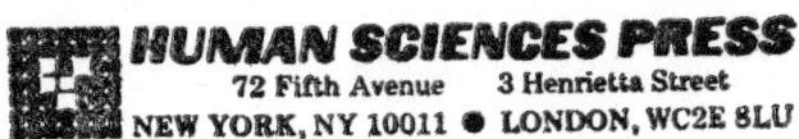

HUMAN SCIENCES PRESS
72 Fifth Avenue 3 Henrietta Street
NEW YORK, NY 10011 • LONDON, WC2E 8LU

Library of Congress Catalog Number 0033-2836
ISBN: 0-87705-333-2

HUMAN SCIENCES PRESS
72 Fifth Avenue
New York, New York 10011

Printed in the United States of America

The Psychoanalytic Review

Vol. 65, No. 1 / Spring 1978

This journal combines THE PSYCHOANALYTIC REVIEW (*founded 1913*) *and* PSYCHOANALYSIS (*founded 1952*). *Former editors of* PSYCHOANALYSIS: *John C. Gustin, Clement Staff. Former editors of* THE PSYCHOANALYTIC REVIEW: *William Alanson White, Smith Ely Jelliffe, and Nolan D. C. Lewis.*

A PUBLICATION OF THE NATIONAL PSYCHOLOGICAL ASSOCIATION FOR PSYCHOANALYSIS, INC.

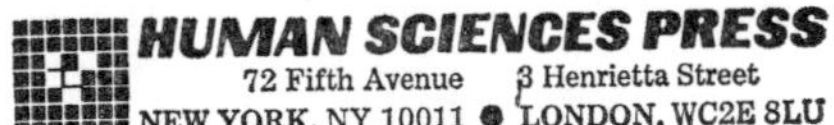
HUMAN SCIENCES PRESS
72 Fifth Avenue, NEW YORK, NY 10011 • 3 Henrietta Street, LONDON, WC2E 8LU

CONTRIBUTORS TO THIS ISSUE

JEFFREY B. BERLIN, PH.D., is a Professor in the Humanities Department of the Philadelphia College of Textiles and Science. Since 1971 he has served as Administrative and Editorial Assistant of the journal *Modern Austrian Literature*. He has published over a dozen studies on Schnitzler, including the book *An Annotated Arthur Schnitzler Bibliography, 1971-1977*.

DONALD G. DAVIAU, PH.D., is Professor of German at the University of California at Riverside and Editor of the journal *Modern Austrian Literature*. His special interest is Austrian literature at the turn of the century, specifically the so-called *Jung-Wien* group. He has published works on Kraus, von Hofmannsthal, Schnitzler, Bahr, Zweig, and Auernheimer.

ADA FARBER, M.A., has taught anthropology and sociology, and has published on Greek myth.

ELIZABETH J. LEVY, M.A., is a teacher of Spanish and German for the Philadelphia Board of Education. She is a member of the Staff Development Group that created the program for teaching about the German Holocaust (1933-1945) in the Philadelphia school curriculum.

THEODOR REIK, PH.D. (1888-1969), born in Vienna and a longt-ime colleague of Freud, served as Secretary of the Vienna Psychoanalytic Society from 1918 to 1928 and came to the United States in 1938. He is best known for his "third ear" approach to psychoanalysis, and his work stresses the primacy of the unconscious in psychoanalytic endeavor.

ALFRED SCHICK, M.D. (1897-1977), born and educated in Vienna, distinguished himself as a teacher and lecturer in Vienna and in the United States and published widely in psychiatry, psychoanalysis, and the psychology of culture. He retired as Assistant Clinical Professor of Psychiatry at the College of Physicians and Surgeons of Columbia University. He was highly identified with Austrian culture, was himself a poet, and knew many literary and political figures of Freud's period. For his cultural contributions to his country he was awarded the Decoration of Honor in Gold for Service to the Republic of Austria.

MURRAY H. SHERMAN, PH.D., is Coeditor of this *Review*. He edited *A Rorschach Reader* and *Psychoanalysis in America: Historical Perspectives*, and is a coauthor of *Roles and Paradigms in Psychotherapy*. He is Chief Psychologist at Jewish Family Service and is in the private practice of psychoanalysis and family therapy.

BERND URBAN, PH.D., is an Instructor at the German Seminar of the University of Frankfurt, West Germany. He has written many essays on psychoanalysis, theology, philosophy, and literature and has edited books and articles on psychoanalysis and the study of literature. Most recently he has written *Hugo von Hofmannsthal and Psychoanalysis: Research and Investigation* (in press).

PREFATORY NOTES: ARTHUR SCHNITZLER AND KARL KRAUS

This Special Issue of *The Psychoanalytic Review* is intended to depict the early development of psychoanalysis within Old Vienna by focusing rather narrowly upon four central figures of that era. The life and work of Sigmund Freud and Theodor Reik are familiar to our readers but this may not be so for Arthur Schnitzler and Karl Kraus. Although Kraus is here represented by only one extensive review article, his significance to the Viennese scene and psychoanalysis merits special attention.

Arthur Schnitzler was born in Vienna on May 15, 1862. His father was a highly successful laryngologist, and Schnitzler himself became a physician with particular interest in using hypnosis to investigate hysteria. While still in his twenties Schnitzler became a member of the Young Vienna group, which included such luminary writers as Hugo von Hofmannsthal, Hermann Bahr, and Richard Beer-Hofmann. In the period 1888-1891 he produced a series of lighthearted plays featuring Anatol, a sophisticated and compulsive seducer of women. Anatol's self-deceptions and megalomania are depicted, as well as the enigmatic and illusory nature of love. These plays and other works received both critical praise and popular acclaim and marked the start of Schnitzler's remarkably productive career as one of Austria's outstanding literary figures.

Although Schnitzler soon gave up the practice of medicine,* his clinical acumen remained conspicuous throughout all his writing. Much of his work focused sharply upon the relationship between sexuality and character—a feature that has often led to his being compared to Freud. Schnitzler was also a sensitive social critic, and

* He continued to provide consultations even into the 1920's. See p. 147.

0033-2836/78/1300-0005 $00.95

certain of his plays dramatized such problems as the chauvinism of the military code of dueling (*None but the Brave,* 1900) and anti-Semitism (*Professor Bernhardi,* 1912). The full breadth of Schnitzler's work cannot be indicated here, but psychoanalysts and clinicians would especially admire *Flight into Darkness* (1931), which gives a compelling picture of the development of psychosis in what amounts almost to an individual case report. *None but the Brave* aroused such fury within military and other circles that Schnitzler was shorn of his reserve commission in the army. Some of his plays so offended the authorities that their performance was banned. Usually the ban was repealed and Schnitzler's popularity increased.

Schnitzler is popularly known in this country for his play *Reigen* (1897), which was twice produced as the movie *La Ronde* in France and several times as the play *Hands Around* in New York. The play depicts the sexual encounters of ten couples who eventually form a full circle of contact. Schnitzler himself had so many doubts about the production of this play that he eventually prohibited its performance, a ban that proved ineffective abroad. He is thus best known here for a play that he did not want produced at all!

Schnitzler's reputation has gone through several cycles. Contemporary criticism was often severe and controversial, and Schnitzler was also subject to anti-Semitic attacks. One review alluded to "the well-known Jewish stink."[14] Nevertheless, from the time Schnitzler started to write until World War I, he was eminently successful in his writing. After 1918 Schnitzler seemed to encounter a kind of writing block and published relatively little. The usual explanation of this rather sudden stoppage is that the Old Vienna that Schnitzler exemplified had come to an end and he had therefore lost both his inspiration and his audience. Some critics believed that Schnitzler's work was centered upon the *süsse Mädel*—the winsomely appealing and freely available Viennese shopgirl of the time. There was no characterization of his work to which Schnitzler objected more vehemently. Schnitzler's innovativeness, his capacity as social critic and depth psychologist, as well as the breadth of theme in his work, all exceed any meanly limited view of his literary stature. Nevertheless, it is probably true that the disappearance of the Old Vienna scene inflicted a wound upon Schnitzler's artistic sensibility from which he did not recover. Perhaps an artist with a broader perspective could have surmounted such a catastrophe.

Schnitzler's personal life was both bountiful and tragic. In his early adult years, which were affluent, he formed many attachments and was perhaps something of a dandy. In 1903 he married Olga Gussman, who was already the mother of his son. Schnitzler's later years were lonely and tragic, partly because of a hearing loss to which he seems to have overreacted. When seen walking alone about the city, he seemed to exemplify the self-absorbed artist quite oblivious to the world around him. In 1928 his daughter committed suicide. Schnitzler himself died October 21, 1931.

At that time the Nazi movement was in its ascendence and German critics dismissed him "as a representative of refined Jewish decadence, and this judgment says basically everything."[13] Although the anti-Semitism passed away, Schnitzler was generally regarded as a writer whose grasp was limited to the Vienna of about 1900. Since the end of World War II, however, there has been increasing critical interest in his work. Comparisons and priorities of discovery vis-à-vis Freud and Schnitzler have appeared in both psychoanalytic and literary sources, which are detailed in Bernd Urban's essay in this issue. There is now an International Arthur Schnitzler Research Association, which publishes the journal *Modern Austrian Literature*. Schnitzler's complex subtleties of plot and theme, his portrayal of role and character, and his social philosophical ideas have been examined. A vital reassessment of Schnitzler has been in progress now for some years.

As early as 1886 Schnitzler attended and reported upon a medical society forum where Freud spoke on the subject of male hysteria, but they did not meet until after a significant exchange of letters in the 1920's. Freud confessed to having definitely avoided direct encounter with Schnitzler out of a fear of meeting his "double," and he asked Schnitzler to keep this remark secret. This letter of Freud is by now quite famous, but Schnitzler's reluctance to seek out Freud has not received attention.

Actually, Freud was more deferential toward Schnitzler than vice versa. Psychoanalysis seemed to Schnitzler both rigid and single-minded in its emphasis upon the Oedipus complex, and the libido theory did not appeal to him despite its core of sexuality. More essentially, however, Schnitzler objected to the tendency of psychoanalysts to read unconscious motivations into his dramatic and literary figures that he had not intended and therefore rather resented.

Furthermore, analysts often interpreted his works as direct exemplifications of psychoanalytic theory, and in fact still do, whereas Schnitzler would have preferred that they be judged on their literary merits alone. Psychoanalysis sometimes seems to detract from literary quality by its reductionistic dissection, somewhat as a joke is spoiled by "explaining" its underlying intent and meaning. However, Schnitzler made no public criticism of psychoanalysis and reserved unfavorable comments to his still unpublished diaries. A far more outspoken critic was Karl Kraus, to whom we now turn.

Karl Kraus was born April 28, 1874, in Jicin, Bohemia, in what is now Czechoslovakia. He was the last of nine children of a prosperous Jewish paper manufacturer, who moved his family to Vienna when Karl was three. Kraus studied German literature, law, and philosophy at the University of Vienna but left before earning a degree.

Beginning in 1892, Kraus published drama criticism and satirical essays in various Viennese periodicals and newspapers. He also made an unsuccessful debut as an actor. In 1899 Kraus founded his own periodical *Die Fackel* (*The Torch*), to which he became the sole contributor from 1911 on. *Die Fackel* consisted of vigorous and biting literary and social satire. It was well known in Vienna, particularly in intellectual groups, and continued in publication until 1936, the year of Kraus's death.

In addition to his satire Kraus produced a large body of poetry and gave popular public readings in which he vividly enacted a number of character roles. At times Kraus appeared as a dedicated misanthrope who attacked everyone and everything. However, he venerated the operettas of Offenbach, extoled Johann Nestroy (a classic Austrian dramatist), and greatly admired Shakespeare, whose work he often presented in his recitals.

Many of Kraus's caustic comments have become classics of satiric wit. When he turned down an enviable position on the *Neue Freie Presse* (the most respected liberal newspaper in Vienna) in 1899, Kraus remarked, "There are two fine things in the world: to be a part of the *Neue Freie Presse* or to despise it. I did not hesitate for one moment what my choice had to be." Kraus despised this newspaper because it tried to combine literary effort with a high profit, and he attacked journalism so bitterly that his name was never mentioned in any of Vienna's newspapers in any context whatever for as long as he lived.

Kraus was especially incensed by careless or even less than perfect use of the German language. He felt that Heinrich Heine (1797-1856), one of the most revered of German lyric poets and writers, had somehow made the German tongue too accessible to the ordinary public. "Heinrich Heine so loosened the corsets of the German language that today every little salesman can fondle her breasts."

However, Kraus's contribution to German literary style was much more than a merely critical one. He was himself an ultimate perfectionist in his writing style, and he incorporated such multiple meanings and unexpected turns of usage as to be considered completely untranslatable until recently. Kraus once commented that he was more concerned that thirty years after his death he be quoted with the correct comma in place than he was in the publication of his complete works. Kraus's lifelong emphasis upon the deepest significance of language is said to have been a direct influence upon the philosophy of Ludwig Wittgenstein (1889-1951), whose work centered upon the basic realities actually created by language itself.[7]

The barbs that Kraus launched so incensed public figures that it was not unusual for him to encounter actual physical assault. He tried in general to avoid being accessible to the public and traveled by auto or airplane in the times before these were popular means of transport. Despite the savagery of Kraus's satire, few people have questioned the integrity or moral seriousness of his work. He was totally horrified by World War I and produced his dramatic masterpiece, *The Last Days of Mankind* (1919), in profound satire of this ultimate folly of men.

Kraus's personal life was also one of persistent protest against convention. He was a sickly child, shy and somewhat disfigured by a curvature of the spine, which may well have contributed to his store of bile. Kraus's mother died when he was seventeen and his father nine years later. Although the family provided a generous income to Kraus, which eliminated his need to earn a living, he separated himself from most of them and at the end of his life requested that they not attend his funeral.

In 1900 Kraus formed an attachment to a beautiful actress who died one year later at the age of 23 and was then vilified in the press. This was an early influence on Kraus's crusade against journalistic opportunism.

Kraus became formally converted to Catholicism in 1911 but left the church in 1923 when he became incensed over his perception of its commercial proclivities. He had been consistently anti-Zionist and even anti-Semitic in his writing, and once said, "Jew boys are the poets of a nation to which they do not belong." However, Kraus's attitude toward his Jewishness should not be oversimplified. As Zohn remarks, "Kraus's convoluted Jewishness is a controversial and ambivalent matter that may be illuminated by paraphrasing Talleyrand's well-known dictum about war: Kraus may have felt that anti-Semitism was too important a matter to be entrusted to anti-Semites."[16]

In 1913, Kraus met Baroness Sidonie Nadherny and fell in love with her. Despite his consistently outspoken opposition to marriage, he proposed several times in the next few years but was turned down by the Baroness, possibly because of class differences. They nevertheless remained intimate friends until Kraus's death.

Kraus continued to be an outspoken critic of society until the very end. His profound belief in his own moral stature is well illustrated by his response to a soft reproach by a close friend when Kraus was on his very deathbed. Kraus suddenly sat up and demanded, "To whom have I ever done an injustice?!" He died June 12, 1936. Bertolt Brecht (1898-1956) commented, "When the age died by its own hand, he was that hand."

Kraus's earliest published reference to psychoanalysis occurred in 1896 and was a positive one, and for some years he remained supportive toward Freud's writings. He perceived Freud as liberal in regard to sexual behavior and used his writing to defend a more tolerant attitude toward homosexuality. Kraus especially praised *Three Essays on the Theory of Sexuality*. At one point, Kraus characterized Freud as another Stanley who discovered the "other dark continent." In the period 1907 to 1908, Kraus became negative and bitter toward psychoanalysis, apparently influenced by Freud's colleagues who wrote psychoanalytically about men of genius. He resented the implications of psychopathology in writers like Strindberg and also attacked psychoanalysis because of its apparent immunity to criticism.[12]

Although Freud and Kraus never met, as far as is known, there was correspondence between them. In 1906, in fact, Freud addressed six communications to Kraus. The most significant was a letter[1a] in which he solicited Kraus's support in defense against Fliess's accusation of plagiarism regarding the theory of bisexuality. At various points in the correspondence Freud praised Kraus for his courage and perceptiveness, requested an opportunity to meet with him, and wrote, "People will praise you for your style and admire you for your wit." The general tenor of the relationship in those years was one in which Freud was courting Kraus because of his influence as editor of *Die Fackel.*[12]

On January 12, 1910, Fritz Wittels (1880-1951), who is best known as an early biographer of Freud, spoke to the Vienna Psychoanalytic Society on "The 'Fackel'-Neurosis," a presentation that emphasized and in fact exaggerated the pathological aspects of Kraus's character.[10] Wittels had earlier been a friend of Kraus and a contributor to *Die Fackel.* Later he became offended by Kraus and turned against him. He seems to have used this meeting of the Society in part to vent his own spleen, as did other members. Freud was tactfully reproachful to Wittels and more balanced in his comments but also remarked that Kraus "lacks any trace of self-mastery, and seems to be altogether at the mercy of his instincts. . . . The most important thing is the clue that by nature [Kraus] is an actor." Freud seems here to be reacting to the fact that Kraus was directed more toward his own emotional catharsis and the violence he was able to stir in others than toward rendering objective truth, and this is perhaps the soundest judgment of all from a psychoanalytic viewpoint. The meeting itself is not one in which analysts today would take pride, but one must remember that it was an early historical moment, long before ego psychology, and at a time when analysts were themselves insecure in their cultural milieu.

Kraus heard about the meeting and its contents, became much more hostile toward analysis than he already was, and attacked psychoanalysis in his most caustic vein. His most renowned aphorism was, "Psychoanalysis is that mental illness for which it regards itself as therapy." He also said that "An analyst turns man into dust," and "Psychology is as useless as directions for using poison." Often he referred to analysts as "psychoanals." However, most telling is Kraus's complaint that psychoanalysts "pick our dreams as if they were our pockets." Kraus resented interpretations of his behavior that may have told him something he did not already know about himself and did not want to know. In that Society meeting Wittels had emphasized Kraus's hatred and displaced attack against his father, and this analysis may have been a barb that struck home.

Freud remained extremely critical toward Kraus. In a letter to Arnold Zweig in 1927, he reproached Zweig for an admiring statement about Kraus "who stands at the very bottom of my ladder of esteem."[2a]

In the writings of Freud there are five scattered references to Schnitzler and also five to Kraus. The most significant is Freud's note in the Dora case,[3] which credits Schnitzler with a knowledge of the importance of resistance (in his play *Paracelsus,* 1899). Freud wrote an admiring letter to Schnitzler soon after this study appeared and mentioned his reference to him.[1b] He later[6] alluded positively to "The Fate of the Baron von Leisenbohg" (1904) as illustrating the taboo of virginity. Reik had published an article in *Imago* in which this same story by Schnitzler was used to illustrate the omnipotence of thought (*cf.* below, pp. 75, 83), and the story has also been analyzed by M. Katan[8] to indicate Schnitzler's intuitive use of the transitional object.

Interestingly enough, three of Freud's five references to Kraus involve the same joke in which Kraus was the subject: "If [Kraus] hears of this, he'll get his ears boxed."[4,5] The ellipsis aspect of the joke implied that Kraus would write so cutting a reaction to what he might hear as to provoke another attack upon him. Freud used the joke to illustrate the technique of wit.

Much of Reik's earliest writing centered upon Schnitzler's work. He researched Schnitzler's very first publications that had preceded the work bringing him fame and also published a book and several articles in which he described the psychoanalytic significance of Schnitzler's writing (below, pp. 69, 75-76, 109-111).

Kraus himself attacked the writing of Schnitzler, as in fact he did the work of most of his contemporaries. Another of Reik's earliest contributions was a one-page parody and counterattack against Kraus's belittlement of Schnitzler. This piece, entitled "The Tiny

Anti-Schnitzler,"[11] repeated the joke about Kraus's ears being boxed, and one surmises that this joke remained in currency over some period of time.

Arthur Schnitzler and Karl Kraus may be taken as emblematic figures of the Old Vienna who interacted significantly with psychoanalysis in its early years. It is to an examination of that interaction that we now turn.

REFERENCES

1. FREUD, E. L. (ED.). *Letters of Sigmund Freud.* Transl. T. and J. Stern. New York: Basic Books, 1960, pp. (a) 249-251; (b) 251.
2. ———. *The Letters of Sigmund Freud and Arnold Zweig.* Transl. E. and W. Robson-Scott. New York: Harcourt, Brace & World, 1970, p. 3.
3. FREUD, S. Fragment of an Analysis of a Case of Hysteria (1905). *Standard Edition,* Vol. 7. London: Hogarth Press, 1953, p. 44n.
4. ———. *Jokes and Their Relation to the Unconscious* (1905). *Standard Edition,* Vol. 8. London: Hogarth Press, 1960, p. 78.
5. ———. Notes upon a Case of Obsessional Neurosis (1909). *Standard Edition,* Vol. 10. London: Hogarth Press, 1955, pp. 227n, 279.
6. ———. The Taboo of Virginity (1918). *Standard Edition,* Vol. 11. London: Hogarth Press, 1957, p. 206n.
7. JANIK, A., AND S. TOULIN. *Wittgenstein's Vienna.* New York: Simon & Shuster, 1973.
8. KATAN, M. Schnitzler's "Das Schicksal des Freiherrn von Leisenbohg." *Journal of the American Psychoanalytic Association,* Vol. 17, 1969, pp. 904-925.
9. KRAUS, K. *Half Truths and One-and-a-Half Truths: Selected Aphorisms.* Ed. and transl. H. Zohn. Montreal: Engendra Press, 1976.
10. NUNBERG, H., AND E. FEDERN (EDS.). *Minutes of the Vienna Psychoanalytic Society,* Vol. 2. New York: International Universities Press, 1967, pp. 382-393.
11. REIK, T. Der kleine Anti-Schnitzler. *Pan,* Vol. 2, No. 40, August 22, 1912, p. 1118. I am indebted to Arno Gruen, who kindly provided the translation of this piece.
12. SZASZ, T. *Karl Kraus and the Soul-Doctors: A Pioneer Critic and His Criticism of Psychiatry and Psychoanalysis.* Baton Rouge: Louisiana State University Press, 1976, pp. 20-30.
13. URBACH, R. *Arthur Schnitzler.* Transl. D. G. Daviau. New York: F. Ungar, 1973, p. 12.
14. WEISS, R. O. Introduction. In A. Schnitzler, *Some Day Peace Will Return.* New York: F. Ungar, 1972, p. 5.
15. ZOHN, H. A Karl Kraus Chronology. In K. Kraus, *In These Great Times.* Montreal: Engendra Press, 1976, pp. 3-8.
16. ———. *Karl Kraus.* New York: Twayne, 1971, p. 41.

In these Prefatory Notes I have drawn heavily from the above works by R. Urbach, R. O. Weiss and H. Zohn.

M. H. S.

THE PLURALISM OF PSYCHIATRY IN VIENNA

Alfred Schick

Why was it in Vienna of all cities that so many discoveries in psychiatry were made? And why was it that around the turn of the century so many participants were of Jewish origin? I explored these questions in a previous paper.[1] Now I would like to illustrate the pluralistic approach, that is, the psychological and organic elements, in the history of Viennese psychiatry. I will interweave historical events with my personal experiences.

The three crowning periods of Viennese medicine coincided with the three heights of Austria's cultural development: the first with the Baroque, the second with the Biedermeier, and the third with "The Moderne."

Basic prerequisites for therapy today are knowledge of a patient's pathological background and of his resulting symptomatology. The endeavors of past periods to define and investigate pathology and symptomatology yielded much. Therapeutic methods used today were relatively unknown formerly anywhere. Therefore, the significance of the well-timed, reasonable advice "Primum non nocere" (Most of all, don't harm the patient) speaks for itself.

The arduous efforts of the Viennese, their courageous and creative minds, were indispensable for the later attempts and success of therapy. Before their time, specific lesions and the seats of pathology were unknown territory. Their search for somatic contingencies dominated the scientific world and made new, effective healing measures possible.

0033-2836/78/1300-0014 $00.95

In Vienna speculation on mind and body dates back to the time of the Roman Empire. *Vindobona* (good wine), the Roman name for the settlement on the Danube which became Vienna, was where Marcus Aurelius recorded his philosophy of stoicism, which contains passages on the major and minor tragedies of life and how to deal with them—calmly and with resignation. His philosophy is echoed by the modern Viennese saying: "The situation is hopeless, but not serious."

Out of the foggy Middle Ages there looms the controversial figure of Theophrastum Bombastus Paracelsus, considered by some to be a cabalist and charlatan,[2] by others a medical reformer. His advocates claim that he contributed a psychosomatic conception that facilitated the development of later medical insights. In furthering his beliefs he dissented from the practices of medieval scholasticism as well as those of archaic, magical medicine. Touchingly, the Paracelsus Society in Salzburg now takes care of his tomb, which is contained in the cemetery where Mozart's parents are buried.

In the eighteenth century Franz Anton Mesmer, a friend of Mozart and dedicated to music, coined the romantic term *animal magnetism*, the force in man that made possible the suggestion and hypnosis of others. His development of this practice was a creative error of great consequence, for it brought into being a new specialty in medicine—psychotherapy—in an age not yet ready to accept it. Like Paracelsus, Mesmer was not taken seriously at first, but in his waning years he became respected by his colleagues.

My familiarity with mesmeric healing in Vienna stems from an episode during my university days. In my third year, before an anatomical lecture, a fellow student called out, "Would you like to earn some money?" I became curious and asked skeptically, "How?" My friend told me that a well-known physician, a *magnetiseur* (a local term), was looking for an assistant in his prospering magnetopathic practice. I visited this physician, and he led me through several lavishly furnished rooms where groups of patients were sitting in comfortable chairs. He demonstrated to me how he interviewed his clients and discussed their troubles with them, always in the presence of other patients. Afterward he touched their hands until they started to shake. In the meantime, with the sick persons' hands shaking, he explained Mesmer's theory and gave them veiled suggestions. Before we parted, he provided me with some literature and lectured about the approach to patients. We agreed on a trial period. I was doubtful of the influence I would have on his patients, but to my surprise I did pretty well and he made me his assistant. A few months later my conscience told me to leave magnetism because it did not go well with the conventional conduct of a physician. However, this experience turned out to be very valuable to my later psychiatric encounters; it taught me the great effect of the therapist's personality on his patients.

Formal medical training began in Austria with the "First Vienna Medical School" during the reign of Maria Theresa and Joseph II. Joseph II, after a visit to his sister Marie Antoinette in Paris during which he was impressed by the hospital Hotel-Dieu, initiated the construction in Vienna of the General Hospital (1784), part of which is still in use, and the beautiful baroque Josephinum for the schooling of military surgeons. Today it houses the library, the reading rooms, and pictures of medical history.* The prominent physicians G. v. Swietan, A. de Haen, Boerhave, and I. P. Frank, a friend of the composer Haydn, were affiliated with the school. Frank, a humanitarian, suggested that the mentally ill not be treated like criminals, but rather as sick people. He saw the importance of public hygiene, introduced the study of forensic medicine, and, most noteworthy, believed that an understanding of anatomical pathology was essential to treatment. It was this era that led later Viennese physicians to derive from anatomical pathology the ills of man, including psychiatric ones.

Another physician, Franz Joseph Gall, stood in the limelight of medical achievements. His *Schaedel-Lehre* (phrenology), namely, the precept that the shape of the skull reveals character traits, was a precursor of the Viennese concept of constitution, for inheritance is carried by matter and biochemical processes. A story goes that Gall was ridiculed in an alliterative pun: *Hier lehrt ein leerer Schaedel leere Schaedel Schaedellehre.* (The study of the skull is taught by a hollow skull to hollow skulls.) Gall described the difference between the white and gray parts of the brain, the crossing of the pyramidal

---

* The historical data are taken mainly from Erna Lesky, *Die Wiener Medizinische Schule im 19 Jahrhundert.* She is the head of the university department of the Institute for the History of Medicine of the University of Vienna.

pathways, and the localization of some nuclei. Most influential were his efforts to discover a connection between physical changes and psychic qualities.

After this period there ensued a temporary state of quiescence for the Vienna Medical School, but by the middle of the nineteenth century another upsurge of medical accomplishments evolved into a "Second Vienna Medical School." This was the *Biedermeierzeit*, the era of great artists in Vienna, e.g., the poet-writers Lenau, Grillparzer, Stifter, Nestroy, and Raimund; the composers Beethoven, Schubert, and the Strauss family; and the painters Amerling and Waldmueller. This Second Vienna Medical School was illuminated by the constellation of the distinguished physicians Karl von Rokitansky, Joseph Skoda, and Ferdinand von Hebra. Hebra laid the groundwork for up-to-date dermatology in his essential book on skin diseases. Skoda stressed realistic clinical observation and the self-healing tendencies of the organism. With his absolute rejection of magical humbug in therapy, he opened the range of vision for the present-day practice of medicine. Rokitansky did investigations in pathological anatomy, including brain pathology. Both Skoda and Rokitansky were excellent teachers, and their influence made Viennese physicians sway, doubt, question, and rely mainly on organic changes, especially pathological anatomy, for the study of all ailments. To quote Erna Lesky: "Viennese medicine became world medicine."[3] From then on the representatives of psychiatry preferred organic explanations in their field.

Among the considerable number of famous physicians who were creators of new medical disciplines, Ignaz Philip Semmelweiss is outstanding in many respects. He already recognized the main cause of childhood fever and advocated asepsis in his publication *Etiology and Prophylaxis of Puerperal Fever*. In spite of the support Rokitansky, Skoda, and Hebra gave him, his revolutionary insight together with his bizarre and paranoic behavior aroused the antagonism of his colleagues in Europe. J. Bauer, in his paper "The Tragic Fate of J. Ph. Semmelweiss,"[4] attributed the progressive decline of Semmelweiss' character and intellectual powers, and his incoherent speeches, to general paresis of the insane. Bauer's conclusion was deduced from clinical impressions and a detailed autopsy report—*Gehirnlahmung* (paresis of the brain), from Rokitansky's Institute of Pathology at Vienna University.

An intense interest in the arts became characteristic of the Viennese physicians, so much so that a great number of them were called *Künstlerärzte*, a local term meaning artist-physician which is still used in Vienna today. To name but two examples, Theodor Billroth, the founder of modern surgery, was one of the best pianists of his time, a composer, music critic, and friend of Brahms; and Arthur Schnitzler was a brilliant master of depth psychology in his fascinating plays and novels. Schnitzler's writings portray Viennese people, their style of life, the beauty of Vienna, the manifold character of Austria's landscape. However, behind the artistic expression the psychologically attentive reader will notice that he implies there exists an inner psychological structure common to all. This universal structure has been a concern of all great artists and thinkers in the past. The relation between art and psychiatry partially explains why Freud and his followers like to analyze artists and the works they created. The qualities of talent and beauty that works of art contain are not, however, accessible to any analytic examination.

Freud wrote a famous letter to Schnitzler, confessing that his evasion of an encounter with Schnitzler had been motivated "by shyness at the thought of seeing my double"—the poet "who found by intuition what I uncovered by hard labor" (May 14, 1922).[5] Another *Künstlerarzt* was Freud himself, who wished to become a writer and indeed achieved a mastery of German prose. For his simplicity and richness of style Freud was honored with the Goethe Prize in Frankfurt, the birthplace of the greatest German poet-writer.

The ambiance of Vienna certainly contributed to the conspicuous union of medicine and art. The multilingual and multicultural Austrian Empire provided the capital city on the Danube with all shades of gifted personalities. Its cosmopolitan atmosphere attracted a steady stream of talents and tales, of lore and literature, of customs and cuisine from all the provinces of the colorful monarchy. In addition, the long tradition of living Baroque, the unique environment, and the passionate love of music and the theater which permeated every stratum of Viennese society were conducive to taking part in the artistic life of the imperial city. The informal meetings of friends and colleagues in the numerous coffeehouses, the crowds filling the concert halls to share enchanting music, the lifelong nearness to humanized nature, and the many surrounding works of art provoked creativity and achievements. Knowledge of history, philosophy, the

Bible, and languages were presumed of the student and specialist in psychiatry. The Viennese psychiatrists instinctively felt that the science of the human mind was connected with the creation of art.

From this atmosphere arose another poet-psychiatrist, Ernst von Feuchtersleben, whose poems we still had to read in public school. Von Feuchtersleben was a friend of two great poet-writers, Franz Grillparzer and A. Stifter. The popular verses with the refrain that I would translate, "It is determined in our Lord's bequest: One has to lose what one loves best," were set to beautiful music by Mendelssohn. Von Feuchtersleben was the first to hold a teaching position in psychiatry in Vienna University. Although inclined to adhere to the philosophical and psychological approach to psychiatry, he considered the union of mind and body. In his best seller *Dietetics for the Soul* he expressed ideas current in psychotherapy even today. Some parts are reminiscent of Marcus Aurelius' stoicism. Latent destructive drives in man were also of concern to Feuchtersleben, so he wanted people humanized and he explained psychic difficulties as a part of social problems, a concept Adler later adopted. At the same time I. Dietl took a purely organic approach to psychic difficulties in his publication "The Anatomic Clinic of Diseases of the Brain." It showed him to be a true follower of Rokitansky's teachings.

Another pupil of Rokitansky was Theodor Meynert, a poet-psychiatrist who was a close friend of the elegiac poet Ferdinand von Saar. Meynert preferred the somatic approach to psychiatry. Under his academic administration the first university psychiatric clinic was established, which became noted for its humanitarian treatment of patients. Meynert reformed and critically examined the topographic anatomy of the brain. He detected locations of the brain cortex that responded to peripheral sensory stimuli. Among other scientific pursuits he elucidated the difference between brain areas conveying associations and the areas conveying sensorimotor discharge.

Meynert ushered in what I would like to call the Third Vienna Medical School, which coincided with the general cultural and economic rise of a predominantly upper middle class in the second half of the nineteenth century. Later, with the ascent of a social democracy that championed the rights of the working class, medical progress continued unabated .

To demonstrate how rich was this period of the third golden age of Vienna, let me mention a few names from the abundance and concentration of creative powers: composers Brahms, Bruckner, Wolf, Mahler, Strauss, Schonberg, and Berg; painters Romako, Klimt, Schiele, and Kokoschka; philosophers Husserl, Mach, Popper-Lynkeus, Wittgenstein, and Buber; architects Loos, Hoffmann, and Wagner; and writers Rilke, Altenberg, Kafka, Schnitzler, Musil, Kraus, Trackl, Broch, Zweig, Roth, Beer-Hoffmann, Werfel, and Hofmannsthal. Berta von Suttner, founder of the peace movement, induced Nobel to establish the peace prize. Then there were others such as Herzl, the founder of Zionism, and Coudenhove-Kalergi, the founder of the Pan-Europa movement. They were all leaders of what the writer Hermann Bahr called "The Moderne." The creative genius of this third golden age contrived new forms of art, philosophy, music, and literature which remain dynamic today. This unique cultural situation spawned creativity in science, the arts, and handicrafts that spread over the world and enriched the cultural evolution of many countries.

In spite of its important technological inventions, Viennese society had a fear of and a contempt for the mechanical world. Franz Joseph I shared with Freud an aversion to typewriting and telephoning and, when possible, even avoided riding in the automobile, which was invented and first constructed in Vienna by Siegfried Marcus.

Therapeutic advances came next in medicine. For example, Holzknecht invented diagnostic X-rays and a method of gauging the strength of X-rays. L. Freund was the first to apply radiological therapy. The science of allergy, introduced by Clemens von Pirquet and Béla Schick, prompted vaccinations against diphtheria, the terror of children and parents, almost eradicating it. Practical surgery of eminent importance for accidents was evolved by L. Boehler. The "saviour" of crippled children, Adolf Lorenz, an orthopedist, invented bloodless corrections of congenital bone malformations to make the patients ready to bear life. A landmark in cardiology was the discovery of mercurial diuresis by Alfred Vogl. Since this discovery innumerable people with congestive heart failure have been rescued from the danger of "drowning in their dropsy." By chance, as a student I had to chart the case history of the patient with whom Vogl made his discovery. Thus I witnessed the process of his careful examination. The old Viennese method of "bedside medicine," blended with keen observation, effected Vogl's success.

Psychiatry built on descriptive symptomatology and underlying pathology needed physicians with scientific qualifications such as intelligence, training, and persistence. Yet, like other medical disciplines, it needed physicians with the endowments of an artist, too—talent, intuition (in Viennese slang, *Kik*), imagination, and the capacity for associative thinking—abilities indispensable for original performance. These two faces of psychiatry separately and rapidly approached each other through clinical medicine, where they gained their fullest expression. Eventually they coalesced, and the united shape turned to the sick with the glance of healing. Psychiatry achieved a culmination which became, along with music, the most striking distinction of Vienna.

In the Vienna of the past, neurology was connected with psychiatry. Even internists such as Chvostek and Schlesinger devoted themselves to neurological practice. L. Tuerck brought new insight into the histology of the nervous system by trying to integrate empirical, physiological, and experimental scrutiny. His research built the foundation for the future growth of neurology.

His successor, Heinrich Obersteiner, built the first institute of neuropathology, which he later donated to the university. The school gained such world renown that physicians from many nations trained at its research center. As *magister magistrorum* Obersteiner had many pupils who became famous in their own right. But Obersteiner did not dedicate himself only to the physiology and pathology of the nervous system. An aspect of the second face of Viennese psychiatry caught his interest—an old and new medium, hypnosis. Schnitzler too was intrigued by it; he used hypnotic experiences in his dramas *Anatol* and *Paracelsus* and wrote a paper entitled "Über funktionelle Aphonie und deren Behandlung durch Hypnose und Suggestion" ("About Functional Aphonia and Its Therapy with Hypnosis and Suggestion") in the *International Clinical Rundschau* (1889). Obersteiner, like Schnitzler, took up Mesmer's healing device. Obersteiner called attention to the hypnotic experiences of Freud and Breuer, who were both fascinated by the therapeutic trance. Obersteiner's most valuable work, however, was his textbook *Anleitung zum Studium des Baus der Nervösen Zentralorgane* (*Introduction to the Study of the Structure of the Central Nervous System*). Again a *Künstlerartz,* he was a gifted musician and conducted Vienna's Physicians Orchestra. After Obersteiner retired, Otto Marburg, who succeeded him, continued somatic psychiatry and advanced the knowledge of brain pathology.

In 1882 Richard Freiherr von Krafft-Ebing took over the psychiatry chair at the university. The pathology of the central nervous system as a basis of clinical consequences was his principal interest. In his interpretation of clinical manifestations defined in his *Textbook of Psychiatry* he expressed and coined new terms such as "compulsive" and "twilight" conditions. A dramatic contribution to medicine was made by his assistant Hirschl, who proved the syphilitic origin of tabes and general paresis, the latter of which was one of the most horrible and deadly diseases of mankind. Hirschl took syphilitic secretions from the primary lesions of recently infected patients and inoculated them into sufferers dying of general paresis. His assumption that they would be immune to a new syphilitic infection appeared correct, because no specifically reactive primary change occurred. When Krafft-Ebing presented this fundamental discovery to a convention of physicians, admiration was general. However, such experiments on human beings were illegal. As the story goes, Hirschl's prosecution resulted in a typical Austrian compromise. His punishment: not being promoted to full professorship. As happens so often in life, problems have not to be solved but survived.

In contrast to the easy-going attitude in Vienna, American reception of Kinsey's statistical investigations on sexual customs in 1948 was rather hostile. About sixty years before Kinsey, Kraft-Ebing wrote one of the first books dealing with sexual aberrations, the *Psychopathia Sexualis*[7] (1886). It did not provoke hostile responses, as did Freud's early psychoanalytic papers. Krafft-Ebing himself criticized Freud's first publications on infantile sexuality. Freud's angry response did not prevent Krafft-Ebing from supporting Freud later in his petition for a professorship. While Freud maintained his belief in infantile sexuality, he revised his theory that sexual advances toward children provoked hysterical symptoms in adults. With his strict adherence to truth, Freud departed openly from his view when he found that the stories of his patients about sexual experiences with a parent or relative were frustrated fantasies. When Freud demonstrated, against all medical expectation, a male with an hysterical feature, he met with opposition in the *Gesellschaft der Arzte* (Society of Physicians). He was so offended that he never again set foot in their building for the rest of his life. But there is no question, as

Johnston writes with astonishing perception in *The Austrian Mind*,[6] that Krafft-Ebing's compilations of sexual data added to Freud's knowledge of psychopathology.

Hirschl's etiological disclosure led to one of the greatest achievements of Viennese psychiatry—the first and only help against a deadly mental disease before the discovery of antibiotics. Organic psychiatry reached its peak with fever therapy for those suffering from "general paresis of the insane," a treatment instituted by the Nobel-Laureate Julius Wagner von Jauregg, a "born clinician." Originally an internist, he was called to take the chair in psychiatry at the University of Vienna, where he followed up case histories of general paretics. Using his genius, he associated the effect of pre-existing febrile afflictions on luetic patients with the keen observation—in the tradition of Rokitansky and Skoda—that general paretics achieved extended remissions after contracting febrile infections such as malaria or erysipelas. After several attempts to generate artificially high temperatures, he successfully chose malaria as the best and easiest way to control fever treatment. He commented upon this method: "We have listened to nature and have tried to copy a course by which nature attains a cure"[3] (my translation).

Furthermore, Wagner-Jauregg's fundamental studies on "Cretinism, Endemic Goiter, and Prophylaxis with Iodized Salt" extended his reputation worldwide. Among his many publications was a work on forensic psychiatry which is still in use. All Wagner-Jauregg's psychiatric innovations were outgrowths of his early clinical training.

In Wagner-Jauregg's time (1875-1940) the other face of psychiatry, the psychological, culminated in the "Revolution in Psychoanalysis." It is historically indicative that Viennese Jews played an incomparably prominent role in psychology at this stage, as they would later. As in a previous period, medicine, especially dynamic psychiatry, once again reached a high point in the midst of a general creative outburst in the sciences, arts, and handicrafts in Vienna (the *Wiener Werkstätte*).

The attitudinal antagonism between the two luminaries of the two aspects of psychiatry, Wagner-Jauregg and Freud, was not as great as some authors made it appear. Both men were lovers of nature and indefatigable walkers. In personal communication, one would perceive that the piercing of eyes of both were tinged with sorrow, although they had a sense of humor and also expressed a liking for trageday. They were classmates and both grew up in humanistic schools in the ambiance of Vienna. Both giants also chose the clinical approach, attaining insight which led to successful therapy. "Clinical medicine" was celebrated in Vienna. The medical doctors in Vienna gained their skill and knowledge at the "bedside." Freud also perceived clinically at the side of the couch or chair the meaning of his patients' free associations. From this emanated his close attention to himself, leading to his self-analysis. Only a few of his very last works are what Freud, in a letter to Struck, called *halbe Romandichtungen* (half novel-fictions).[5]

Freud was a connoisseur of literature and poetry. Expressions of weariness and foreboding color some of his letters and work, as they do Austrian literature generally. The psychotherapist and the poet, the musician in the vineyard and the composer of genius, were bewitched by the theme of love and death, and likewise Eros and Thanatos were main motifs in Freud's vision. The Viennese tendency to ruminate on the ephemeral quality and complexity of life's mysteries has its roots in the Baroque era, whose attitudes and ideas have continued to pervade Austria's culture and affected both Freud's and Wagner-Jauregg's perception of human existence.

Wagner-Jauregg may have demonstrated a deference to Freud by promoting his assistants Heinz Hartmann and Paul Schilder to professorships. As head of a university department, Wagner-Jauregg had autonomous power, yet he let these coworkers teach psychoanalytic theory and practice. In their later years Freud and Wagner-Jauregg exchanged letters of mutual regard and friendship on their birthdays.

Freud, trained by Meynert and the famous physiologist Ernst Wilhelm von Brücke (1819-1892), started his medical career in neuropathology. Brücke, an artist and a specialist in Renaissance culture, brought into being the new medical specialty of physiology. Of Freud's many papers in the somatic sphere, the study "Zur Auffassang der Aphasien" (1891), his last in neurology, has special value. Freud was aware that his psychological discoveries did not unravel the ultimate etiology of neurotic or psychotic ailments, but rather added understanding to the motivations of human behavior. One can sense Freud's view from his repeated statements such as, "The man with the syringe is already right behind us," or, "*Als ob die Einsicht in seelische Mechanismen die Kentnis des Zugrunde liegenden Chemis-*

mus ersetzen Konnte" ("As if the insight into the psychological mechanism could replace the knowledge of the basic chemical make-up"), from his letter to A. Lipschütz, 1931.[5] All this is a precursor of Einstein's theory of the interchangeability of matter and energy under certain conditions. Thus Freud, like Wagner-Jauregg, believed in a biochemical etiology of mental ailments. Wagner-Jauregg made an outstanding contribution to the organic approach in psychiatry with the fever therapy of general paresis. Freud also made significant contributions in neuropathology and, in addition, called attention to the anesthetic qualities of cocaine, thus inspiring the invention of local anesthesia. According to his own assertion, he had wanted to use this discovery in his practice, as his colleague Carl Koller in fact did.

While Wagner-Jauregg opposed hypnosis and demonstrated his opinion that it was inefficient by a risky experiment, Freud opened up a new dimension through his genius and courage by investigating the free association of the hypnotized. Josef Breuer focused Freud's attention on a method for the psychological exploration of hysterical symptoms and wrote with Freud *Studies on Hysteria* (1895). In this work Freud declared: "I decided to use Breuer's method to investigate [Emmy von N.] under hypnosis. It was my first attempt at using this therapeutic method."

Breuer, the son of a teacher of Jewish religion, was at one time an assistant to Johann von Oppolzer, a cardiologist whom Breuer ranked among the group of pioneer physicians in Vienna. As an internist, Breuer uncovered the function of the labyrinth of the ear and the nervous mechanism that controls normal breathing. Breuer shied away from pursuing hysteria to its conclusions, however. Though in Vienna there was not the Victorian prudishness that characterized the American approach to life and sex,* Breuer seems to have feared that he would harm his thriving medical practice, which comprised the cream of Viennese society, if he revealed the sexual pathology behind hysteria. Breuer refused to accept an esteemed academic position offered to him in Vienna, explaining that due to his time-consuming practice a professorship would be too much of a burden to him. Besides, Breuer was a brilliant musician and devoted many hours to this pleasure. Brahms, Brüll, and other celebrities participated in his highly acclaimed chamber music recitals.

---

* See Freud's letter to James J. Putnam, July 8, 1915.[5]

What shocked Vienna most, however, was not so much the sexual revelations of psychoanalysis as the transfiguration of the traditional image of man. Freud dethroned the human race from its fictitious position of rational supremacy and undermined narcissistic illusions by his disclosure of the unconscious motivations in human conduct. Among Freud's most sarcastic opponents were the two brilliant Viennese writers, both of Jewish origin, Karl Kraus and Egon Friedell.

What happened to Freud in the controversy over his "new wave" of science brings back to my memory the derision suffered by other celebrities. For example, Francis Joseph I had to intervene on behalf of, and defend against intrigues, the exacting Jewish director of the Vienna Court Opera, Gustav Mahler, who deserved only praise for the new style of his compositions and his mastery as a conductor of singers and orchestra, a mastery which elevated one of Vienna's musical centers to a height of unsurpassed fame. One of the greatest contributors to the glory of the *Haus auf der Ringstrasse*, as the opera house was called, was Richard Strauss, who had to leave his post because of the difficulties he encountered with his coworkers and critics.

Grumbling was a favorite pastime among Viennese citizens, whether citizens by birth or by choice and inclination, and they grumbled especially about their seductive city, which they loved so much. Freud, typically Viennese, also tended to ignore or minimize the achievements which in fact existed all around him. Despite their complaints, important Viennese rarely moved away, no matter how attractive the offers they received. Freud remained in Vienna, ignoring all the favorable opportunities he had to move to other cities. Only self-preservation forced him finally to leave the city. L. Frank, the daughter of *Hofrat* Frankfurter, director of the university's library, told me about her father's last visit to Freud. As a young girl she had accompanied her father to say good-bye to the great man. It was a sad meeting. Pointing his arm to the window, Freud had said, with moist eyes, *Und das muss ich alles verlassen* (All that, I have to leave), meaning Vienna.

Considering man's psychological makeup at the turn of the century and the fact that a Catholic monarchy was in power, one marvels at the Austrian tolerance toward Freud and his teachings; in another place the master would have been burned at the stake, at least symbolically. In the United States in 1909 Morton Prince faced a court action for "obscenities" because he published a psychoanalytic paper in his *Journal of Abnormal Psychology*. Prince was saved from a lawsuit only because of his status as a former mayor of Boston.[10]

Through many years Freud could afford to live comfortably in a big household with a servant. He first achieved recognition in Vienna when he was awarded the *Stipendium*, a grant to study abroad which was given to very few. Many years later he was awarded the honorary citizenship of Vienna, which was personally presented to him by the Lord Mayor, Karl Seitz, a popular and distinguished figure. Freud was generous: he paid for Reik's analysis in Berlin and helped to support Lou Andreas-Salomé when she was in need after Hitler came to power in Germany. In fact I myself am indebted to Freud for saving my life by allowing the use of his name on my behalf when Hitler persecuted the Jews in Austria.

Freud dedicated most of his time to his unique work, but he had other interests, too. He enjoyed valuable relics and read books on archeology; he also read widely in world literature and philosophy; he was fluent in a number of ancient and modern languages. During his best years, Freud could afford expensive travels and vacation resorts, as well as visits to conventions. He accepted his painful and fatal illness with resignation and heroic patience.

Freud's disciples made consequential contributions to psychoanalysis, spreading their master's doctrine worldwide, especially after the Nazis forced them to emigrate. Of the many émigrés of personal merit and professional rank Theodor Reik gained special attention in America. In Vienna he had represented a living link between Freud and Schnitzler.

In a captivating paper Murray Sherman called attention to Reik's "worship" of Freud.[11] It happened that Freud and his pupil liked and quoted the same nonpsychoanalytic authors, such as one of the greatest satirical dramatists in world literature, the Viennese actor Johan Nestroy. Furthermore, Reik treasured about fifty pictures of Freud, which covered the walls of his living room, and he mentioned Freud's personal advice conspicuously often.[11] In fact, Reik imitated Freud's habit when he named his son Arthur after Schnitzler, for Freud also gave his children the names of people he admired. Reik told me that when he took leave of Freud the latter remarked, "People who belong together do not have to be glued together."

Other followers of Freud turned from his methodology to establish their own psychological theories and therapeutic techniques. One apostate of Freud, Alfred Adler, stressed the sociocultural element in the etiology of mental distress. Adler's *Individual Psychology* (1919) influenced all later schools of social orientation. His terms "style of life," "social feeling," and "organ inferiority" became, like the terms Freud coined, a part of everyday thinking and language, so that many who use them today are not even aware of their origin.

Like Freud, Adler benefited from the humanistic education characteristic of the Viennese style of life. He also had the stamina to climb mountains, a popular hobby in Vienna. In contrast to Freud, Adler was inclined to an epicurean outlook and could enjoy the gifts of life, though his cheerfulness was occasionally subdued by somber moods. I used to see him sitting in the courtyards and gardens of Vienna under the flower-candles of chestnut trees or blooming lilacs, sometimes with the famous logopedist E. Fröschels, a poet, sipping new wine to the accompaniment of the *Schrammel Quartet* (this wine and music are specialties of Vienna). Adler loved the coffeehouse and instructed his followers there.

The investigations and conclusions of these Viennese pioneers profoundly influenced and modified many disciplines, such as pedagogy, anthropology, sociology, criminology, and medicine, and permeated the whole literature. Freud's daughter Anna and Adler's daughter Alexandra continued in their fathers' footsteps. Under the influence of Adler, Aichhorn, and Anna Freud—the pathfinder of child psychoanalysis—community psychiatry began. J. Tandler, world-renowned professor of anatomy and commissioner of health in Vienna, one of the giants of that time, reformed civilization with a new social approach to health and welfare.[12] His work was copied all over the continents, and much of what is now accepted as a matter of daily life was first planned and executed by him. We owe to Tandler the establishment of the first vocational guidance and psychotherapy clinics and the first marriage and childbirth counseling offices; he even instituted genetic counseling. Alexandra Adler, a member of Wagner-Jauregg's university department, identified and described the centers of convergence of the eyeballs and the pupils in the midbrain and was the first to call attention to the psychology of accident-prone industrial workers.

Like her father's concept of organ inferiority, Alexandra's brain research linked a psychological approach to somatic psychiatry, as did Freud's grounding of instincts in a biological origin. According to Freud, Goethe was the first to use a chemical analogue—Elective Affinities—to characterize the mutual attraction of certain persons. Freud borrowed the very word *analysis* from chemistry for his new investigations.

Another dissenter from Freud's theories was Wilhelm Stekel. A superior violinist and poet, he innovated a simplified psychoanalytic treatment in his *Technik der analytischen Psychotherapy.* Stekel and his leading pupil, Emil Gutheil, practiced "psychoanalytic psychotherapy," which seems to be the most often eclectically applied form of psychotherapy today.

Among the outstanding scholars in Wagner-Jauregg's institute, a few should be mentioned. Berze occupied himself with clinical descriptions of schizophrenia. My excellent teacher Erwin Stransky recognized the dissociation of personality in schizophrenia before Bleuler's description, calling it "intrapsychic ataxia." Besides investigating neurological problems, Stransky wrote about manic-depressive disorders and advocated psychic hygiene at a time when no one else was thinking of it. His *Textbook of Special Psychiatry* (1904) is in many respects still useful. E. Sträussler advanced psychiatric histology and contributed to the question of heredity in neuropathology. Even the radiological interpretation of skull and brain diseases was started in Vienna by A. Schüller, whose name has been attached to the Schüller-Christian syndrome. The first physician to diagnose the Western sleeping sickness, encephalitis lethargica, was Constantin von Economo (1917). He found the center of sleep regulation and published a standard work, *Die Zytoarchitektonik der Hrinrinde des erwachsenen Menschen* (*The Zyto-Architecture of the Brain Cortex of the Adult*).

Otto Pötzl, who began as Wagner-Jauregg's assistant and later became his successor, excelled in the research of brain pathology, in which he combined aspects of both psychoanalysis and Gestalt psychology. His consequent interpretation of the interaction of brain functions made him a pioneer of a dynamic approach to brain activities. Modern electrobiological experiments demonstrate the truth of his insights.[23] Pötzl created a new procedure in psychiatry by attempting to integrate the clinical symptoms, psychology, and brain pathology of well-defined cases. His lectures to prepare students for their psychiatric examinations were of extraordinary vivacity, wit, and clarity. He probably absorbed these qualities from his father, whose weekly stories, published widely in newspapers and journals, were full of humor and spirit. Last, the memory of J. Gerstman will live on through the Gerstman syndrome, a condition consisting of finger agnosia, acalculia, and agraphia.

In the same cultural period, the sociopsychological orientation was taken up by I. Moreno. He inaugurated group sessions and, motivated by the city's involvement with the theater, called his therapy "psychodrama." He introduced the "encounter" (*Begegnung*) into the psychiatric vocabulary in his publication "Invitation to an Encounter."[13] Meanwhile, at Wagner-Jauregg's institute Sackel introduced the first physical remedy for a functional psychosis—insulin shock. Many physicians, more or less analytically oriented, received their psychiatric experience and training under Wagner-Jauregg: e.g., Erwin Stengel, Heinz Hartmann, Ludwig Eidelberg, Hans Hoff, and the Adlerian Rudolf Dreikurs. Dreikurs was one of the first group therapists. All of these men settled later in the United States.

The most eminent of Wagner-Jauregg's assistants was Paul Schilder, a member of the Viennese Psychoanalytic Society. He embodied the two faces of psychiatry in a masterful way. Like many of the aforementioned psychiatrists, he expanded somatic psychiatry. He described a hitherto undiagnosed cerebral pathology which has since been internationally named Schilder's disease. In his career, Schilder rounded out the trend of the Vienna psychiatric school by enumerating a multiplicity of causal factors—hereditary, physical, psychological, and sociocultural—in psychiatric etiology. He related physiology to psychology and ethical philosophy and re-evaluated hypnosis, anticipating practically everything being said today about it. Schilder provided valuable information to almost all areas of neurology and pathology. His most valuable book, according to his own judgment, was *Das Körperschema* (*The Image and Appearance of the Human Body*, 1923),[14] in which he stated that our body's image is a kind of mental design that we develop in our physical selves as we grow. It is a representation of our body as a whole and of each organic component according to its situation, form, texture, and action; each part is distinct, yet they are interrelated. One example of the body's image is the so-called "phantom limb" sensation of amputees: the phantom limb is felt as reality. Although Schilder stressed the importance of Freud's dream interpretation and libido theory, he believed "that life is not directed toward the past but rather toward the future; that psychological processes are directed toward the real world of continuous trial and error." Gestalt theory and Adler's "individual psychology" were combined in his work *Gedanken zu Naturphilosophie*.[14] Under Schilder a new area of psychiatry developed in Vienna: psychosomatic and somatopsychic medicine. Schilder proved himself to be one of the originators in the integration of psyche and soma, considered in connection with the environment. The biological makeup and life experiences of the individual, according to Schilder, mold the form a psychosomatic ailment takes.

In 1930 Schilder accepted the invitation of the psychiatrist Adolf Meyer to move to New York. He became Associate Professor of Psychiatry at New York University Medical College and Director of the Psychiatric Department of Bellevue Hospital. He also organized the Schilder Society in New York, of which I have had the honor of being president. Schilder died in 1940, run over by a car after a visit to his wife and new-born daughter.

As a principal proponent of psychosomatic medicine, Schilder repeatedly stressed his belief in the future of psychopharmacology. His work precipitated the acceptance of somatic psychiatry and chemical therapy to such an extent that Vienna became a center of psychosomatic medicine.

Constitutional makeup, I believe, is a psychosomatic entity in personality formation. J. Bauer noted the influence of constitution in 1917. Freud once wrote to Ludwig Binswanger, "Constitution is everything" (*Anlage ist alles*),[16] and in a letter to E. Voigtländer, Freud affirmed the significance of heredity.[5] In Tandler's opinion, the physical and psychic fate of man was decided at conception. In collaboration with Bauer and others he published a journal, *Zeitschrift fur Konstitutionslehre*. Freud agreed with Bauer's original conviction of the importance of heredity in mental disturbances. He defined *Anlage* as a potential which is determined like a blueprint at the moment of fertilization.

This view of constitution implies an inborn potential for inadequate reaction to stress or even an inability to cope with the usual demands of human development. Such "organ inferiority" is more intrinsic to the etiology of psychiatric disorders. Environmental agents specify only the manifestation of the *Anlage*. The personality structure results from inherited and experienced components. Bauer, a pioneer in the elucidation of the clinical import of constitutionis, established a "psychosomatic" clinic within his department of internal medicine at the Polyclinic in Vienna. In this hospital I observed a peculiarity in the elucidation of the clinical import of constitution,[15] established the sick persons referred as sufferers of neurasthenia or hypochondria often revealed a traumatic experience that had precipitated their complaints. In addition, their histories showed a cyclic occurrence of the "illness," which reminded me of the periodicity in depressive conditions. Furthermore, in many cases their symptoms repeated themselves in a stereotyped way and with almost photographic exactness. When I questioned them, I was frequently able to uncover a hereditary ingredient consisting of depression in blood relatives or a pyknic habitus. This induced me to believe that the physical pains had an underlying emotional pathology. The follow-up on these cases sometimes showed the emergence of manifest depression, occasionally many years later. Some patients, operated on repeatedly, continued with the same symptoms. Interrupted by Nazi terrorism, I resumed my investigations at the Vanderbilt Clinic in New York, adding conviction to my impression that such patients were depressive without depression, so in 1947 I published "On a Physical Form of Periodic Depression."[17] The surprising success of antidepressive medication has since corroborated my opinion. An assistant in Bauer's internal medicine department, Max Schur, Freud's personal physician, published a remarkable psychosomatic study "On Insufficiency of the Anterior Lobe of Hypophysis."

In the psychosomatic sphere, both R. Heilig, a brilliant internist, and Hoff initiated a striking series of experiments to prove the interaction of soma and psyche long before the word *psychosomatic* was known. In one of these projects, they generated herpes labialis by suggestion in persons who had previously reacted with herpes after frightening events. The herpes fluid thus made available was inoculated into the cornea of rabbits and caused an eruption of specific blisters.[18] The experiment of Heilig and Hoff demonstrates how the organism's psychic and physical expressions are influenced by the surrounding world.

In another project, the two researchers watched radiologically the movement in the gastrointestinal tract of patients under hypnosis. Alternately cheerful and stressful suggestions resulted in corresponding changes in the secretion of gastric juices. Biochemical comparisons of gastric juices yielded differences between relaxed and tense patients.

Oswald Schwarz published the first systematized volume on psychosomatic medicine, *Psychogenesis and Psychotherapy of Physical Symptoms.*[19] In his preface Bauer examined "The Individual Constitution as Basis of Nervous Disturbances."

Conversely, Joseph Wilder, an erudite scholar, emphasized "somatopsychic" pathology. He described how mental symptoms can obscure or precede a somatic illness. For instance, an inherited trend of obesity may be hidden by a neurotic syndrome or affective complaints may be prodromal to a later manifest multiple sclerosis. Psychic phenomena produced by hypoglycemia were noticed for the first time by Wilder. He also wrote in detail about the possibility of ingesting chemical substances to induce neuroses or psychoses. As director of a well-known neurological institute in Vienna, he let neurotic cases stay in the hospital for constant observation and therapy. This practice was new in medicine.

In recent years the pluralistic schools, having recovered from their decline during Hitler's terror and World War II, have reemerged with a new two-sided presentation of psychiatry and a reorganization of the neuropsychiatric university department. Besides his scientific and teaching competence, Hoff turned out to be a capable organizer. He had to emigrate and arrived in New York via Baghdad. For some time we practiced together in the consultation service of Columbia Presbyterian Medical Center. After the liberation of Austria, he accepted the chair of psychiatry at the University of Vienna. During one of my visits there I saw Hoff and he invited me to go on a sight-seeing tour of his newly created psychiatric installations, a few buildings of which were sprinkled in the Vienna Woods.

Thus I became acquainted with an institution for asocial and criminal adolescents; a rehabilitation center with workshops, one for schizophrenics and another for drug addicts; and a self-sufficient homestead for alcoholics. I saw one especially innovative therapeutic undertaking. At Hoff's suggestion, heavily guarded confinement had been reserved for inmates found to be unmanageable in the ordinary prison wards. Hoff looked after each of these "patients" and supervised the therapeutic efforts of his assistants. The *Herr Professor,* as he was called with respect by the convicts, effected with an unobtrusive skill a benevolent transference and elicited the same in return. Such treatment took place in a remote room, purposely without protection or prison personnel nearby. Generally, techniques of different psychological schools were applied. Feeling a bit ill at ease, I was introduced by Hoff to every single prisoner who entered this "office," from murderers to arsonists. Names were politely mentioned and handshakes exchanged. It was the last stop of our rounds. Then my friend drove me back to my hotel. Hungry and tired, I washed my hands, thinking of Lady Macbeth, who could not clean off the bloody spots of murder from her hands.

In addition to Hoff, there were three other men of stature who assisted in the rebirth of Vienna's psychiatry. Konrad Lorenz, a biologist and former professor of comparative psychiatry, was the founder of an institute of behavioral research (*Verhaltungs forschung*). From observations of animal behavior he and his pupils (especially Otto Koenig) evolved a concept that he termed "culture ethology." By this he meant that the development of the structure of the central nervous system and its consequences are determined by the "ancestral history" of adjustment to a particular environment. When the environment changes, no longer necessitating a certain conduct, remnants perpetuate themselves as symbols, ornaments, or implements of a social function. Lorenz's much discussed book *On Aggression* deals in an original way with such sociocultural attitudes.

V. Frankl, the developer of existential psychoanalysis, considers the absence of a realization of a meaningful orientation in life the decisive factor in the formation of a neurosis. He does not, however, completely exclude the roles played by Freud's biological and Adler's sociocultural concepts in the growth of neurotic conditions. According to Frankl, positive values are essential for the well-being of man; they form the primary base for his spiritual existence. Existential analysis sees human life directed by the need to find sense in his personal existence, expressed by a striving for values. Therefore, one has to investigate and make the individual conscious of the significance of his being, awakening a feeling of relationship and responsibility to society. Every period produces a specific type of psychotherapy. Its relativity to place and time is especially obvious in Frankl's teachings. His method of analysis grew out of his way of surviving in a concentration camp;[20] nevertheless, it should not be minimized. In certain cases it can be very helpful. Frankl also developed a group therapy technique which, in typical Viennese manner, he called "logodrama."

Walter Birkmayer and his coworker O. Hornikiewicz delved into the somatic effects of Parkinson's syndrome with its affective aberrations. They analyzed the brain tissue of dead Parkinson patients and found a grossly decreased amount of Dopamin. They concluded that the etiology of Parkinson's disease may be due to the diminution of Dopamin. Accordingly, they used L Dopa as a therapeutic substitute in Parkinson's disease cases, as insulin is used for diabetics. The amazing result confirmed Birkmayer's expectation. Not only did the physical condition of patients improve; their depressive states, common among sufferers of Parkinson's disease, lessened, allowing them to seek social relationships and thus escape their unavoidable loneliness.[21] In all probability, L Dopa or its derivatives will turn out to be of therapeutic importance for neuroses and psychoses.

At present psychopharmacological remedies have proven to be extremely useful in psychiatry. The days when Wagner-Jauregg would lecture that every depression took its course by nature, no matter what treatment was applied, are gone. Gone also is the validity of his dryly humorous quips; for example, his remark, alluding to the ebb and flow of a depression, "The last physician is considered the best." However, we are still far from integrating the diverse components distinctive in the Viennese pluralistic approach: physicians' speculation, philosophical doctrine, sociocultural influence, interpersonal relationships, constitution, physiological and psychodynamic occurrences, and the source from which psychiatry in Vienna came forth, pathological anatomy. The multifaceted diagnostic and therapeutic advances in Viennese science suggest that little in contemporary psychiatry and neurology has not had its foundation in Vienna.[23]

P. Brenner, the current head of the Vienna University Division of Psychiatry, recently spoke in New York, and I participated as an invited discussant. During the lecture I learned from him that the psychiatric and neurological clinics are now separated and divided into a psychotherapeutic / depth-psychological department and an institute for experimental research.

In this essay I have tried to describe the pluralistic approach to psychiatry in Vienna. Common to all schools there have been an attempt at intuitive perception of diagnosis and an individualistic psychosomatic understanding of man. The representatives of this clinical medicine, living in a baroque culture, were *Künstlerärzte* in the original sense of the term. At the least, they displayed a common interest in the arts and nature. People of different nationalities and faiths in the great Danubian empire have taken part in the unfolding of this colorful medical canvas. A past to remember, a future to create.

NOTES

1. SCHICK, A. The Vienna of Sigmund Freud. *Psychoanalytic Review,* Vol. 55, No. 4, 1968-1969.
2. MOOK, F. *Paracelsus: Eine kritische Studie.* Wurzburg: Staudinger, 1876.
3. LESKY, E. *Die Wiener Medizinische Schule im 19 Jahrhundert.* Graz: Bohlers, 1965.
4. BAUER, J. The Tragic Fate of J. Ph. Semmelweiss. *Calif. Med.,* 1964, pp. 98-264.
5. FREUD, S. *Letters 1873-1939.* Ed. E. L. Freud. Transl. T. and J. Stern. New York: Basic Books, 1960.
6. JOHNSTON, W. M. *The Austrian Mind.* Berkley: University of California Press, 1972.
7. KRAFFT-EBING, R. *Psychopathia Sexualis: Eine klinisch-forensische Studie.* Stuttgart, 1886.
8. ROBERT, M. *La Revolution Psychoanalytique: La Vie et l'oeuvre de Sigmund Freud.* Paris: Poyot, Collection de l'Homme, 1964.
9. BREUER, J., AND S. FREUD. *Studies on Hysteria.* New York: Avon, 1966.
10. JONES, E. *Das Leben und Werk von Sigmund Freud.* Bern: Huber, 1960.
11. SHERMAN, M. Freud, Reik and the Problem of Technique in Psychoanalysis. *Psychoanalytic Review,* Vol. 52, No. 3, 1965.
12. SCHICK, A. The Life and Work of Julius Tandler. *Pirquet Bulletin of Clinical Medicine,* Vol. 16, 1969.
13. MORENO, L. *Die Gottheit als Komediant.* Vienna: Anzengruber, 1911.
    ———. The Viennese Origins of the Encounter Movement: Paving the Way for Existentialism, Group Psychotherapy and Psychodrama. *Group Psychotherapy,* Vol. 22, 1969.
14. SCHILDER, P. *The Image and Appearance of the Human Body.* New York: International Universities Press, 1950.
    ———. *Uber das Gelbstbewusstsein und Personlichkeitsbewusstsein.* Berlin: Springer, 1914.
    ———. *Gedanken zur Naturphilosophie.* Vienna: Springer, 1928.
15. BAUER, J. *Konstitutionelle Disposition zur Inneren Krankheiten.* Berlin: Springer, 1921-1923.
16. BINSWANGER, L. *Erinnerungen an Sigmund Freud.* Bern: Franke, 1956.

17. Schick, A. On a Physical Form of Periodic Depression. *Psychoanalytic Review,* Vol. 34, No. 4, 1947.
18. Helig, R., and H. Hoff. Die Psychische Entstehung des Herpes Labialis. *Med. Klinik,* pp. 1302, 1928.
———. Uber Beziehungen zwischen Houtreaktivitat und Ovarialfunktion. Klin. Wochenschrift 4, 868, 1925.
19. Schwarz, O. *Psychogenesis and Psychotherapy of Physical Symptoms.* Vienna: Springer, 1925.
20. Frankl, V. *From Death Camp to Existentialism.* Transl. E. Lasch. Boston: Beacon Press, 1959.
21. Birkmayer, W. Ten Years of L Dopa Therapy of the Parkinson Syndrome. *Wiener Klin. Wochenschrift,* No. 13, 1971. Birkmayer, Bernheim and Hornikiewicz. Biogen Gehalt in Verschiedenen Hirnsegionen, 1961.
22. Brenner, P. *Lecture in N.Y.C. History and Modern Developments of Austrian Psychiatry,* 1973.
23. Hoff, H., and F. Seitelberger. Die Geschichte der Neurologie und Psychiatrie in Wien. *Wiener Mediz. Wochenschrift,* 1966.

The Psychoanalytic Review
Vol. 65, No. 1, 1978

ON THE EFFECT OF UNCONSCIOUS DEATH WISHES*

Theodor Reik

Translated by Harry Zohn

EDITOR'S INTRODUCTION

In Fragment of a Great Confession *(1949) Reik refers at some length to the following article, "On the Effect of Unconscious Death Wishes," translated here for the first time. He indicates how the article had explored certain obsessions and compulsions that had assailed him in 1913, the time the article was written. Reik uses the concept of unconscious death wishes to explain these symptoms, and the article thus marks the very beginning of his lifelong preoccupation with death wishes in their various guises. The piece has considerable biographical relevance in amplifying the information provided by Reik in* Fragment *and also is illustrative of psychoanalytic writing in its early moments.*

Reik, at the age of twenty-five, had already published more than twenty articles in applied psychoanalysis, but this essay was his first clinical piece. At the time "Unconscious Death Wishes" was written, Reik had not yet formally begun psychoanalytic practice. He had been with the Vienna Psychoanalytic Society since November 15, 1911, when he presented "On Death and Sexuality" and was unanimously voted in as a member. The "patients" he describes below are frankly introduced as friends and acquaintances, and it is likely that he himself is one of the individuals analyzed in the latter portion of

* Reprinted from the *Internationale Zeitschrift für ärtzliche Psychoanalyse,* Bd. 2, 1914, pp. 327-353.

0033-2836/78/1300-0038 $00.95

the essay. Although the article was published anonymously, Reik could easily have been identified by his colleagues through the personal data included, such as the fact that Reik's father was a railroad inspector. Reik's efforts at disguise were often halfhearted and rather transparent. It is likely that the two sisters described as Erna and Mary (pp. 597) were Reik's fiancée Ella and her sister Mary and that the chatting episodes with Daisy (p. 55) were later described as liaison with Vilma in Fragment *(pp. 81, 83-84).*

Schnitzler receives special attention in the article. Reik uses some dialogue from The Vast Domain *(1911) to illustrate his concept of death wishes (p. 58 fn.) and he reveals that his reading of* The Big Wurstel Puppet Theater *(1905) was the central day remnant behind a death dream about his father (p. 53).*

The article is also significant in its mention of self-punishment symptoms (pp. 58, 65), since this is an early forerunner of such work of Reik as The Compulsion to Confess and the Need for Punishment *(1925) and also* Masochism in Modern Man *(1940). In addition to the experience of suffering under the burden of his own compulsions, Reik was also influenced here by Freud's "Fragment of an Analysis of a Case of Hysteria" (1905), where he alluded several times to the theme of self-punishment. Freud's article may have influenced Reik to choose the name Dora (the pseudonym Freud chose for his patient) as a pseudonym for Ella, soon to be his wife. The title of Freud's essay may have figured in Reik's much later selection of* Fragment *as a title. This influence of Freud upon Reik remained conspicuous throughout Reik's writing. Nevertheless, it is important to note that where Freud later developed the idea of self-punishment into his theory of the death wish, Reik did not follow him but remained with self-punishment/masochism as sadism turned inward against the self.*

This early article by Reik is intended, in part, to be read in conjunction with the one that follows (pp. 68-94).

—M. H. S.

Then Job answered and said, Even today is my complaint bitter: my stroke is heavier than my groaning. Oh that I knew where I might find him; that I might come even to his seat! I would order my cause before him, and fill my mouth with arguments. I would

> know the words which he would answer me, and understand what he would say unto me. Will he plead against me with his great power? No; but he would put strength in me. There the righteous might dispute with him; so should I be delivered for ever from my judge. Behold, I go forward, but he is not there; and backward, but I cannot perceive him. On the left hand, where he doth work, but I cannot behold him: He hideth himself on the right hand, that I cannot see him.
>
> —Job 23:1-10

PREFACE

In the dreams and fantasies of psychoneurotics psychoanalysis has been able to uncover death wishes directed against admired and beloved persons, and it has explained them on the basis of the ambivalent emotional characteristics of these patients. But so far little attention has been given to the great role which death thoughts and death wishes play in the emotional life of healthy persons. This is true as well of the disguises and distortions habitually employed by such trains of thought to avoid betraying their dangerous cargo. My essay is intended as a contribution toward the filling of these two lacunae.

Most of the following analyses were made on a person whose mental health I have no reason to doubt—that is, myself. It would be petty if we analysts refrained from the analysis of our own death fantasies after our master and some of his pupils have published interpretations of their own dreams. The personal sacrifice appears small compared with the profit which could accrue to research from such reports. It is to be hoped that the intellectual interest of the reader in these complex problems will lead him to forget that the person analyzed is the analyst himself.

ANALYSIS OF SOME COMPULSIVE THOUGHTS AND ACTS

My father died on June 16, 1906, of arteriosclerosis. This heavy blow, which I later perceived as the most momentous in my life to date, plunged the eighteen year old into severe emotional conflicts. Their point of departure was the rejection of a feeling which arose in me on the day my father died. The beloved man sat in an easy chair breathing heavily and groaning. Two physicians were at his side, and I was sent to the pharmacy to get what was needed for an injection. I was well aware of the importance of this assignment, for the doctors had left me no doubt that this was the remedy of last resort. While I was running through the streets as fast as I could, I suddenly fantasized that my father had already died, leaving me as the head of the family and the protector of my mother and my sister. The wishful nature of this fantasy was clearly indicated by the feeling of satisfaction that accompanied it. Another indication of this was the fact that I stopped running and started walking fast; the excuse I made to myself was that I was out of breath. I sought to suppress my evil thoughts, and I ran all the more quickly as if to make atonement. I arrived home in a state of near collapse. My father was lying dead on a sofa, and all I remember is that at this sight I was stunned as if by a powerful electric shock and threw myself in front of the body in despair.

The next days were filled with grief and mourning over the passing of my dear father. I was tormented by an increasing longing for his familiar face and his kind words. In those days I often asked myself what I would have given if he could have gone on living. At first my answer invariably was: my own life. But later I rejected this trade with the sophistical argument that such a sacrifice could not appease my longing for my father, and the stake was decreased further and further until I was obliged to realize that I was not willing to give up even one year of my life to bring him back. Despite all my longing for him, I did not quite manage to suppress a certain satisfaction at being allowed to replace my father when at the age of eighteen I had to take care of important family matters. To my great consternation, a powerful wave of sexual excitement swept over me in those days of mourning, an excitement that consciously had no definite object. I fought it with all my might, but it was in vain; my sexual drive was so great that three days after my father's death I sought and found a transition from the (infrequently practiced) masturbation of my puberty to normal sexual intercourse. These sexual acts, which I did not understand and condemned with disgust, were followed by severe self-reproaches which took approximately the following form: Now that your father, this noble and beloved human being, is dead, at this very time when all your thoughts should be of him, you do such ugly things. My sexual drive, however, was stronger than my will, and each act of sexual intercourse was followed by a period of remorse, anxiety, and contrition. I must confess that in those days I shuddered at myself. Although I did not *consciously* believe in immortality and a life after death, I could not rid myself of the thought that my dead father in his last hour knew about my death wish as well as about my sexual activity, and that he despised me and would punish me. I feared in particular that my deceased father would punish me by letting me become ill and eventually die, and this is why I was especially tormented by the possibility of venereal disease.* At the same time I was wracked by doubt whether I could not have kept my father from dying if I had run faster that evening. Such guilt feelings beset me especially when I had to laugh heartily at a good joke or a clever phrase. Immediately I reproached myself for being able to be so cheerful such a short time after my dear father's death. It is obvious that in those days I was already at that stage which usually precedes the manifest eruption of an obsessional neurosis. Nor was the counter-struggle lacking; to avoid being in those good moods which invariably were paid for with severe self-torment, I increasingly curtailed my social life. During my years in secondary school I had certainly not been among the most diligent students; but now I tackled my studies with undreamed-of zeal and worked from early morning to late at night. This far-reaching protective measure had the schismatic nature of neurotic symptoms. It served to combat temptations (sexuality, cheerfulness) and at the same time was self-punishment for my egotistic desires, but it also revealed my repressed complexes. The ambition that animated me in those days was the result of a desire to surpass my father, and my self-chosen solitude was, as it were, an indication of autoerotic sexual activity. The work which I did so stubbornly while neglecting all *joie de vivre* clearly bore the mark of penance. It was a concise expression of my ambivalent attitude toward the deceased. My ambition not only contained a concealed desire to surpass my father, but it also served as a safety valve for my affection for that irreplaceable man. Work was to make me worthy of him and prove to him that he had not lavished his sacrifices and concerns on an unworthy person; it was intended, so to speak, to rehabilitate me in his eyes. Since my father was dead, this last intention might appear strange; but it may be explained by a superstitious thought, one vainly fought by my

* The same mechanism was at work in a case of compulsion neurosis (fear of infection) the development of which I was able to observe closely.

conscious, that my dead father knew about my career and was "inspecting" it, as I told myself at the time.*

My distress had reached its zenith when I became acquainted with the teachings of Freud. It is to them that I owe my liberation. Now I was able to discern in my desires and doubts a special coinage of universally human emotions, recognized their connection with the formation of psychoneurotic symptoms, and no longer viewed myself in isolation as a criminal and depraved type. The ethical influence of the physician on the patient, which the Zurich School misses in the traditional technique of psychoanalysis, is inherent in the elimination of the "splendid isolation" of neurotics. Once such neurotics recognize their sexual and hostile impulses as universally human ones, they no longer regard themselves as rare criminal types. Anyone who has ever heard a neurotic complain about his being different knows that the patient perceives this as a heavy burden. Self-analysis showed me that my death wish on that errand to the pharmacy was an expression of my ambivalent attitude toward my father. I was able to explain to myself my sudden onrush of libido as well with the aid of analogies: the death of my father removed the inhibitions which had hitherto blocked my choice of an object (originally my mother).† All I consciously remember is that my father always discussed sexual matters with me in an open and natural way. Yet in my early childhood it must have been he who prohibited sexual activity (masturbation). The aftereffects of that prohibition were the

* As I realized later, this term, too, had a psychic basis. My father was a railroad inspector. On visits to his office which I had made as a child, I had received a lasting impression of the magnitude of his sphere of power by observing the behavior of his subordinates.

† A modern poet, Rainer Maria Rilke, once expressed a similar mood: "In solchen Nächten wissen die Unheilbaren: / wir waren . . . / Und sie denken unter den Kranken / einen einfachen, guten Gedanken / weiter, dort, wo er abbrach. / Doch von den Söhnen, die sie gelassen, / geht der jüngste vielleicht durch die einsamsten Gassen: / denn gerade *diese* Nächte / sind ihm, als ob er zum ersten Male dächte: / lange lag es über ihm bleiern, / aber jetzt wird sich alles entschleiern / und dass er das feiern wird, / fühlt er . . ." (In such nights the incurables know: we were . . . And among the patients they continue thinking a simple, good thought from where it broke off. But of the sons they left behind, perhaps the youngest will walk in the loneliest streets; for precisely these nights make him feel as though he were thinking for the first time. For a long time there was a leaden weight on him, but now everything will reveal itself, and he feels that he will celebrate that. . . .)—From *Das Buch der Bilder,* Part Two, "Aus einer Sturmnacht," V.

unconscious roots of my remorse over my sexual intercourse ("belated obedience").

In later life I had to feel with increasing intensity the great and indeed decisive force of my ambivalence toward my deceased father. As I struggled to gain my independence and a livelihood and as I realized how great the difficulties were and how small my energy to overcome them, I increasingly realized the importance of being alone. Emotionally I perceived this loneliness as "being left alone," and in many an hour of despair I leveled reproaches at my dead father. What I said to myself was this: He should not have died so soon and left me lonely. Who will now help me in my struggle for existence? He was weary and *wanted* to die. But it was his *duty* to go on living, at least until his children were provided for. Absurd though these thoughts were, it was hard to suppress them. It is plain that my independence was a weak reed. The current of hostility which placed the stamp of reproach on this reasoning was closely bound up with a current of affection. The loss of my father had depressed me; it was hard to do without him.

In connection with the flaring up of my libido after the death of my father, I should like to refer to the analogous jubilation of savages after the killing of the totemic animal, the animal which Freud's analysis identifies with the father.* The sadness at the death of the totemic animal is the prelude to the festive joy which appears as a "permissible, even prescribed excess, a festive breach of a prohibition."

A mysterious incident of recent days has given me an opportunity to get a better understanding through analysis of my death wishes against my father and the ensuing moods of remorse and penance, matters which I have previously regarded as closed.

The girl I intended to marry had contracted a serious illness (pneumonia), and I had visited her in her summer home at N. I was planning to return to Vienna on a certain train. Considerably behind schedule, I started out for the station, which was about a half-hour from the villa of Dora's parents. As I was walking along, my thoughts understandably were on Dora's illness, which worried me a great deal. Suddenly I had the following idea: *If I don't go to K. to be with my sister, Dora will die.* This idea gradually became so com-

* Cf. Freud, "Die infantile Wiederkehr des Totemismus," *Imago,* August 1913.

pelling that near the N. station I turned around and headed for K. (three-quarters of an hour from N.), where my sister was spending the summer. I vainly tried to make myself understand the absurdity of my compulsive idea; I was afraid that what I feared would happen if I did not carry out my plan. As I attempted to realize what deeper reasons were motivating me to visit my sister, I remembered a letter which I had received from her a few days previously. As I was able to veryify at home, she had written as follows:*

Dear Brother:

I forgot to tell you that on June 29 we must kindle a *yahrzeit* light for Papa.† If you like, I shall leave a light burning for you as well, but then you should come out on Friday so you can be present at the kindling. If you don't come, then I'll count on your kindling a light yourself. Go to the synagogue, too.

With kind regards.

Irene

—Wouldn't you like to visit the cemetery some day?

My analysis must start with this letter, for it makes possible a first revision of the form of my obsessional idea. In the form in which the compulsive connection occurred to me, a connecting link was missing which might have contained the most important thing and for certain reasons might have been withheld from my conscious thinking. The actual formulation of my apprehension was as follows: *If I don't go to K. and don't hallow the memory of my father by kindling a light there, Dora will die.* How did it happen that this interpolation, and thus the real reason for my visit to my sister, remained concealed from me? Upon receipt of her letter I had felt annoyed. I dislike being reminded of my duty, because I believe that I do it almost too conscientiously. Then, too, I am not pious enough to believe that kindling a light has more than a symbolic significance. The postscript to Irene's letter in particular was food for gloomy

* I was going to throw that letter away after I received it. My keeping it was determined by the unconscious processes revealed by analysis. Thus this involuntary preservation constitutes a symbolic act (reminder of my duty).

† In accordance with the precepts of the Jewish religion, members of a family kindle an oil light in memory of a deceased relative on the anniversary of his death.

thought. To my sister I had often expressed my view that true piety consisted not in conventional visits to graves and the observance of religious ceremonies but in living in the spirit of the deceased dear ones. I had definitely decided not to visit Irene on that day, but now my decision was voided by my obsessional apprehension. It shows that despite my conscious conviction I unconsciously do ascribe real significance to the kindling of *yahrzeit* lights. What seems strange is that the memory of my father, who could not have known about my relationship with Dora, was connected with Dora's illness. Once I had reached this point, my thoughts returned to my visit to Dora. It is necessary to give details about it here. Dora received a peculiar education from her father. From her early childhood, age three, to her twentieth year she was not allowed to go out in the street alone or speak with a man, nor was she permitted to go to the theater or attend a dance, a party, etc. Her father hated the idea of marrying off his daughter; he would not hear of it. He would have placed the greatest obstacles in the path of my relationship with Dora and an engagement to her. Thus we had only two options: avoid any meeting or exchange of messages for years (for even Dora's letters were subject to paternal censorship) or keep our relationship secret from her father. We chose the latter course of action, and it was prompted by the fact that Dora's father was frequently away on trips and that I could meet my beloved then. We had to wait for a more propitious period when we might accomplish our union without consideration for the father's veto. We took Dora's mother into our secret, and after a hard struggle she had to decide to join us in our "deception," because Dora threatened that she would otherwise leave her parental home for good.

My animosity against Dora's father mounted steadily. When I visited Dora during her illness, her father was not there. I could not contain myself any longer and in very strong language expressed to my future mother-in-law my anger and indignation at such an abnormal situation. Dora's mother, to be sure, was hardly to blame for the unnaturalness of the family situation, but she was there, and in my excitement I did not discriminate. Still, to avoid hurting the good woman even more, I had to suppress what was troubling me most of all. This concerned Dora's father, who translated his absurd theory about the general moral inferiority of women into practice by incarcerating his daughter from early childhood on, thus concealing his own incestuous fixation behind educational reasons. In this connection it is easy to understand that very intensive death wishes against that man emerged in me and even penetrated into my consciousness. Thus I can relate a daydream which occupied me frequently and very pleasurably. I fantasized a situation in which I would no longer require the consent of Dora's father to our union. I saw myself in his study, asking him calmly and self-confidently for Dora's hand. I imagined that a phrase I had often read in novels as a boy would be his answer: "You are a nobody and have nothing." My daydream put the following ridiculous response to this rejection in my mouth: "Of course, this is none of your business, most honored sir [*Verehrtester*] (*sic*). But I think it is important for you to know that it would give me the greatest pleasure to bash your head in with the books which I have already written." This truly bloodthirsty fantasy is surely amusing in its stupidity, but it seems significant by virtue of the tendencies—particularly my death wishes against Dora's father—for which it served as a point of breakthrough. In its presumptuousness it also shows my overestimation of myself. The quantity of my books here substitutes for their value; it is supposed to show my importance in its true light. The fact that I want to actualize my death wishes specifically through my books shows that the humiliation which I constantly experience at the hands of Dora's father (though without his knowledge and intent) is what weighs most heavily on me.

My hostile attitude toward Dora's father was hardened even more by the serious illness of the beloved girl, for I gave him some of the blame for it. Immediately after the first symptoms of the illness appeared he should have sent for a doctor—not the local doctor who was treating Dora at the time (and whom I consciously esteemed highly), but an outstanding internist from nearby Vienna. Inwardly I reproached him with wasting money on his private amusements and taking only half-measures to save money when his daughter's life was at stake. That these preposterous accusations are explainable only by the intensity of my emotions is shown by the fact that Dora's father was away on a trip and did not even know about his daughter's illness. My excitement was heightened even more by the prospect that he would return in a few days and that I would then not be allowed to visit Dora, get no news of her condition, and would suffer all the torments of uncertainty. This apprehension brought me back to my critique of the abnormal situation in Dora's family. If her father were healthy (and not, as I believed, a severely neurotic person), I could visit her openly and in his presence and keep informed about her condition.

All these thoughts must have been unconsciously at work on my way back from N., for in analysis they came out in an onrush of associations. The insults directed at Dora's father which I was not permitted to utter and my evil wishes for him constitute a large part of the psychic material for the development of a subsequent compulsive idea. As we have seen, I had directed similar wishes against my father, too. It seems as though these have been transferred to a father substitute; my father and Dora's father play a similar role as disturbers of my love life. There was another factor that promoted the unconscious identification of the two men. In my excitement I had threatened Dora's mother that I would induce Dora to leave her parental home if the unbearable conditions there were not removed. When the mother asked what Dora, who had no means of her own, would then live on, I had proudly answered that they should let *me* take care of that. When I had calmed down, I had to realize that I have neither property nor a secure position that would enable me to keep my promises. My self-confidence had been utterly out of place there. With some bitterness and shame I realized once more that my present situation hardly permitted me to think of marriage, and the thought that in the near future there was no prospect of improvment depressed me. Once again that chain of reasoning included the reproach that my father had left me too soon and that he ought to have helped me. I had sometimes found my dependence upon him oppressive, which also applied to Dora's father, and early on I had made repeated attempts to rely on my own strength and shape my own life. These attempts, too, increasingly convinced me that my energies were not sufficient and that I needed his help.

My death wishes were directed against Dora's father and regressively followed the path of old childhood feelings against my own father who had once impeded my sexual activity in the same way. The consecration of his memory as symbolized in obsessional thinking by the kindling of a light now appears as penance, as a begging for forgiveness for the evil wishes directed against him. There still remains the task to explore the psychogenesis of this linkage: If I don't go to K., Dora will die. The psychoanalytic investigation of the compulsive thoughts of neurotics shows that such expectations of misfortune always constitute psychic reactions to evil wishes, and this is true in my case as well. The unconscious process is reflected as follows: Because I have wished death for Dora's father (and mine), he will take revenge by depriving me of the one I love most. I must placate him by doing my religious duty which proves my respect and love for him. A necessary premise for this is the unconscious assumption that my father knows about my wish and my expiation, and this was shown in my superstitious fear shortly after his death. To me this case seems to be a striking confirmation of the parallel which Freud drew between "compulsive acts and the practice of religion" (*Kleine Schriften zur Neurosenlehre,* Vol. 2), because here the content of the compulsive idea is a religious ceremony and enables one to derive it from the same mechanism of protection compulsion. The kindling of lights is tantamount to a reconciliation with the father; it is a sacrifice intended to prevent him from avenging himself on me for my evil wishes against him. It is significant that this sacrifice is accomplished precisely through the kindling of a light—that is, the confirmation of my death wish. This compulsive act furnishes an individual analogy to the psychogenesis of sacrifice in religion.*

> The importance which sacrifice has gained quite generally resides in the fact that it offers the father amends for the outrage committed against him in the same act which perpetuates the memory of this outrage.

No one who is familiar with the complexity and overdetermination of psychic processes will be surprised that in the analysis of this obsessional idea it was possible to reveal still other feelings as determinants of its formation. One of the main factors which would seem to make Dora's father's consent to marriage between us impossible is his fanatical anti-Semitism which has assumed the most absurd forms. Dora's mother is an aposate from Judaism.† After a period of indifference to my fellow Jews I became increasingly more interested in Jewry and its strangely tragic destiny. Psychoanalysis

* Cf. Freud, "Die infantile Wiederkehr des Totemismus," *Imago,* 1913.

† Here I venture to hypothesize that the anti-Semitism of persons with neurotic tendencies is due in large measure to a transference of hostile feelings from their closest relatives (father, wife, etc.).

taught me why this interest emerged during my father's illness and gained in intensity after his death.* Once I had even found myself considering leaving the Jewish fold—not only to remove in this way the obstacles in the path of my union with Dora but also to secure for myself in this reprehensible manner all sorts of other opportunities for my career. I immediately rejected this notion, but it seems to have continued in me unconsciously. It is precisely this area of nationalistic tension that is the conscious source of my hatred of Dora's father, and this seems to make a meeting of the minds with him impossible. This is what enabled me to fixate the hostile feelings which I had toward him as a father substitute on his anti-Semitism, while I bestowed my affectionate feelings upon my father and the Judaism that he represented to me. Thus the fulfillment of my religious duty and piety (kindling of lights) is also an acknowledgment that I belong to my people, and as such it is an expression of defiance against Dora's father. Thereby, so to speak, I make my father and myself the promise that I shall never be disloyal to Judaism, of which I consider myself an integral part, and that I shall never deny my father and my Jewish origin, not even if this stubbornness were to mean the loss of Dora.†

There was also a topical occasion to concern myself with the religious-nationalistic complex of Judaism. (The expression "religious complex," which is often misused, should be regarded with great caution here. For precisely this case, more than most others, seems designed to demonstrate that an individual's attitude toward religion constitutes merely a psychic deepening and widening of his relationship with his father and not, as Dr. Stekel assumes, an independent, separable area.)

In my abovementioned conversation with Dora's mother she had pointed out that according to the Jewish tradition, too, it was

* In our time, the younger generation has found a way within this relationship to create two discrete objects for the ambivalent attitude meant for the father. The deprecatory and antagonistic tendency now is directed against the religion, which is regarded as obsolete and superfluous, while the affectionate and delicate current flows toward the Jewish people to which the young Jewish generation in Western countries adheres with great pride (Zionism, Jewish nationalism).

† It seems to me that the attitude of a modern Jew toward his people and his religion is determined most of all by his relationship with his father. This is particularly true of the intensifying interest of an individual in his people which manifests itself as he grows older. It goes hand in hand with certain typical changes within the father complex and with the psychic revaluation brought about by the transformation of filial feelings into fatherly ones.

a sin to alienate a daughter from her parents.* In response I hastened to assure her that under such unusual conditions I found it necessary to deviate from my usual views. For the rest, I reminded her of an injunction in the Bible according to which a wife should leave her father and mother and go with her husband.†

When I had arrived at this point in my analysis, memories of my mother emerged in me. At first she regarded my relationship with Dora as one of the necessary follies of youth; later she noted that I was serious, and then she became interested in Dora. The girl called on her a few times, and my mother assured me that she liked Dora. It seems significant to me that on Dora's last visit my mother gave her a hearty kiss. At that time my mother already was in the first stage of the illness that was to carry her off. A few days before her death I had a conversation with her which later I frequently remembered as though it had been rife with presentiment. We spoke about my older brother who was leading a miserable, joyless bachelor's life and even then displayed clear symptoms of a severe neurosis. My mother expressed the view that the real reason for his cheerlessness was his failure to marry, his having "missed the boat." I asked: "Then I should marry young?" She answered: "Yes. And you have already found the right girl." Thus Dora was, as it were, given my mother's blessing. My mother's spontaneous approval was now added to the outward and inward similarities which bound Dora and my mother together and unconsciously determined my choice of object. On the day of my mother's passing, at the time of the poor woman's death-struggle, Dora came to our house. This visit appeared like a fateful sign: my mother passed away gently, and by way of consolation I now received a younger successor on whom I could bestow my love.

---

* The argument of Dora's mother seems to have made some impression on me, for I gladly took the earliest opportunity to refute it anew. Soon thereafter I read an old Jewish folk song and hastened to send it to my future mother-in-law with a reference to her harangue. The first stanza of the poem, which is entitled "Liebeslied eines jüdischen Mädchens" (Love Song of a Jewish Girl), delighted me with its warmth and naturalness. It goes something like this: "Ich will laufen durch alle Gassen / und will schreien: 'Wäsche waschen!' / Brot mit Wasser will ich essen, / *Vater und Mutter will ich vergessen,* / wenn ich nur kann bei dir sein" (I will run through all the streets and cry, "I take in laundry!" I will eat bread and water, *I will forget my father and my mother* if only I can be with you).

† I am fully aware that unconsciously I tendentiously distorted the Bible words.

These memories of scenes long believed forgotten gave me the key, so to speak, to the most hidden chamber of my obsessional ideas: I had identified Dora with my mother, just as her father represented my own father to me. My impulses and fears regressively go back to an old childhood constellation: my incestuous affection for my mother, my death wish directed against my fatherly rival, and the fear of the consequences of this wish, the expectation of misfortune. In my compulsive idea a certain antithesis is established between Dora and my father. This antithesis corresponds to the vacillation between a female and a male as love objects.* For alongside the hostile current against my father, the opposite psychic tendency also comes to the fore—particularly in my reverence for my father's memory and my fear that Dora will die, a fear that conceals an unconscious wish in the same direction.

But the wealth of associations in my obsessional idea still does not seem to be exhausted. A further overdetermination results from my feelings toward my sister Irene. She had reminded me to come to her home and perform an act of filial piety. After my father's death I had resolved to be helpful to my younger sister and to watch over her until I could relinquish this duty to her husband. But it was impossible for me to keep this unspoken promise; in fact, in recent months some circumstances obliged me increasingly to slacken my relationship with Irene. One of the main reasons for this was that dividing my interests conflicted with my love for Irene. For without being willing to admit it, Irene was intensely jealous of Dora, who was depriving her of her brother's love, and she was not strong enough to suppress the manifestations of this antipathy. With the supersensitivity of a young girl to whom the loss of her parents had meant the loss of her greatest love objects, who did not have the love of a man as a substitute and now was to be deprived of the love of her brother by a "stranger," she regarded every expression of my affection for Dora as an indication that I was neglecting her. Even though my conscious reflection sought to devalue such reproaches as unjustified and exaggerated, unconsciously I must have recognized their justification, for the associations to my compulsive idea which now emerged left me no doubt that I was feeling remorse

* Compare a similar relationship in the patient in Freud's basic essay "Notes upon a Case of Obsessional Neurosis."

at my neglect of Irene. Though I did not admit it, I regarded her reminder of my duty toward my father as a reminder of my duty toward *her,* a duty which I had so selfishly neglected. This is another source of my feelings of guilt and responsibility toward my father whose memory had prompted me to vow to take care of Irene. My fear that my father would punish me by making Dora die is rooted as well in the unconscious realization that it was precisely because of Dora that I had not done my fraternal duty. From this angle, too, the ceremony of kindling a light appears as an expression of my guilt feelings and my moods of remorse as well as an attempt at expiation.

The psychic congestion caused by my death wishes was not fully eliminated, because it still affected my dream of the following night.* This is what I dreamed: *I was asleep. The door opened and a man came in and approached my bed with slow, strangely heavy steps. He wore muttonchop whiskers, and there was a dead serious expression on his face. I noticed that he was wearing a clown's costume which was out of keeping with his generally serious mien. He kept coming closer.* (The rest is blurred.) I woke up with a pounding heart and feelings of fright. Some striking features of this dream I was immediately able to trace back to known factors. That slow, ponderous gait reminds me of my father, who was rather corpulent, and so do the muttonchops. The "dead serious" expression, too, I often observed in him, with painful emotion, in his last days. In the dream the meaning of the adjective is that he really is dead, that in fact he is Death.† The clown's costume is determined by my reading of Schnitzler's profound and cheerful burlesque *Zum grossen Wurstel.* I had been reading this work on the evening of that eventful day in order to relieve myself of the pressure of my sad thoughts (of Dora's illness, my uncertain future, my anger at Dora's father, and my longing for my own father). I remember that the figure of Death which at the end of Schnitzler's one-act play changes into a clown made a great impression on me (connection with the day). For me there was no doubt that the dead man in my dream was supposed to represent my father. Only after struggling with great obstacles was I able to realize why the beloved man wore such

* This is another confirmation of Freud's rule that dreams contain the real text and meaning of compulsive ideas.

† Artists, too, depict Death as a dead man.

striking garb—something that I had observed with astonishment in the dream. In frequently interrupted associations I remembered many scenes from my early childhood in which my father had poked fun at himself and revealed to us his small, all-too-human weaknesses with exaggerated candor and in an effort to give us pleasure.

But as a child I must have taken my father's merry self-presentation quite seriously, because it diminished my respect for my father, gave sustenance to my hostile currents, and provided a conscious rationale for them; they were rationalized. Thus it happened that I was often afraid that other people, too, would recognize my father's weaknesses. I was always concerned that he might commit some act of clumsiness, be caught with his guard down, etc. (It is obvious that this anxiety derived from a repressed wish.) There is no denying it: I must confess that sometimes I was ashamed of my father, that high-minded and irreproachable person, and only reluctantly accompanied him on his walks.* We now recognize how the dead man of my dream got into the clown's costume; the return of the infantile material was manifested in that feature. The absurdity of the dream image is the reflex of my infantile scorn of my father.† Well, what did my dead father want of me? He wanted to take me away with him and kill me. This explains my anxiety during the dream: the deceased takes revenge for my having wished his death as a child (which for a dreamer and a neurotic coincides with the murder itself) by killing me. The dream is based on the unconsciously operative *lex talionis.* Its whole structure, which is the structure of the typical dreams about burglars, shows the infantile roots of my death wish against my father: the threat of castration because of childhood masturbation. The expectations of misfortune in my obsessional idea and in my dream have the same motivation.

Earlier I stated that these analyses refer to a person who in general enjoys good mental health. Still, I will not deny that I have noticed in myself certain "neurotic attitudes," to use Dr. E. Hitschmann's excellent term. I believe, however, that the borderline between mental health and mental illness is so fluid that any person who has grown up in the present cultural milieu with a certain

* Observation of many children has taught me that such infantile feelings of embarrassment relating to one's father are of frequent occurrence.

† Cf. Freud, *The Interpretation of Dreams.*

"psychosexual constitution" (Freud) will have occasion to relate similar things about himself.

An incident which also occurred in the days when I was worrying about Dora once more brought home to me the great dynamic force of unconscious processes. When Dora's illness was supposed to reach the crisis stage, I had the following idea when coming home one evening: *If I chat with Miss Daisy today, Dora will die.* Miss Daisy is the daughter of my landlady who was in the friendly habit of chatting with me on some evenings, something that I always regarded as an unwelcome interruption of my work. In the wake of my compulsive idea there immediately arose in me the impulse to lock the door to my room (a safety measure in the literal sense). My analysis did not proceed from this incident, but from the ensuing tormenting feeling of jealousy. In the light of Dora's whole character, with which I had been acquainted for years, this emotion was completely without foundation, and it was all the more absurd because I knew that Dora was now in bed, seriously ill, with a high fever, and under the care of her parents. Self-analysis had often taught me that the endopsychic perception of one's own erotic temptation which is unconsciously projected onto the love object is one of the most significant psychic roots of jealousy. My analysis of the compulsive connection which I established between my conversations with Miss Daisy and Dora's condition was able to base itself on this insight. My fear, whose meaning was obscured by the elliptical distortion technique, actually is as follows: If I cheat on Dora with Miss Daisy, Dora will die. I must have taken an unconscious liking to my *filia hospitalis* [landlady's daughter], whom, on a conscious plane, I tended to dislike. The death wish that lurks behind my obsessional idea is directed against Dora: the faithfulness which I owe her prevents me from having any relationship other than a conventional one with Miss Daisy and obliges me to overlook the advances she is making toward me. That is why I wish Dora were out of the way. There is also a memory that serves to locate the unconscious connecting links in the formulation of my compulsive idea. Dora had once written me a letter in which she told about one of her dreams: She caught me red-handed with another girl and cried out to me: "I can't bear this; I'm going to jump into the Danube!" My fear made reference to this memory; in its restored form it goes like this: If I cheat on Dora with Miss Daisy, Dora will take it so much to heart that she will commit suicide. The primary purpose of the safety measure of locking my door is to protect me from myself, from my sexual temptation. This, after all, is the purpose of all protective measure, even those taken by compulsive neurotics. They are supposed to protect the patients from the power of hostile and sexual desires which they reject as incompatible with the requirements of civilization and the moral demands of the self.

As may be seen from this example, jealousy was fully developed in me.* Another compulsive idea also originated from the strong emotions aroused by this jealousy. After Dora's recovery, the two of us visited my sister and met a number of young ladies and gentlemen there. During a discussion of a general subject I expressed an opinion that differed from the views of those present. My chief opponent in the debate was a young man whom the girls regarded as especially "nice." My dislike of him as well as his objections to my views forced me to defend these by adopting the most extreme and most paradoxical positions; as a result, all those present united against me. Even Dora rejected my position with words of reproof. It now seemed to me that the formulation of her views indicated a certain harshness toward me and a leaning toward my opponent. I ended the discussion testily with a witticism that was as forced as it was cheap.

That evening I accompanied Dora from K. to N. and en route tried to tell her what I felt: that my exaggerated jealousy fastened on her opposition to me and made me draw conclusions from it (unjustified ones, as I consciously realized). The shortest route to N. was over a hill called the "Black Tower." It had already turned dark, and after saying goodbye to Dora I felt mildly afraid of taking the path, lined by thick shrubbery, via the "Black Tower" where I thought all sorts of shady characters hung out at night. I therefore planned to choose a more frequented roundabout route through the town. As I approached the ascent to the "Black Tower," the following compulsive idea emerged in me: *You must go via the "Black Tower."* I vainly tried to oppose to this my mounting fright and feeling of dread. After I had safely completed my walk, I realized that this compulsive act was supposed to constitute a sort of divine judg-

* At this point I need only indicate that this jealousy was conditioned by my strong repression of homosexual currents.

ment. This is how I reasoned: *If Dora remains faithful to me, nothing will happen to me on my walk. But if she becomes unfaithful, I shall be attacked and stabbed to death.* As regards the second alternative, I sought to remove from it all the repugnance arising from my fear by telling myself that life without Dora's faithfulness would have no value for me in any case.* As one can plainly see, the compulsion I felt was secondary—an attempt to compensate for my doubts about the faithfulness of the beloved girl. The transferability of these doubts is shown by the fact that the abovementioned alternative was modified by me along the way. Since there were no signs of an attack upon me, I imagined the following possibilities of decision: If I don't encounter any suspicious person of whom I would have to be afraid, Dora will remain true to me; if I do, she will become unfaithful. As chance would have it, I did meet a man toward the end of my walk, and since I am very near-sighted I bumped into him in the darkness.† In a flash the question that I was allowed to pose to fate changed as follows: If this man gets rough with me, Dora is unfaithful; if he places no obstacles in my path, she is faithful. The man very politely begged my pardon and went on his way. In fact, I can say that my encountering him subsequently removed my fear of that sinister road. But now another doubt emerged: Did I feel fear during that encounter? Was the man suspicious to me? May I regard my encounter with him as a decision? I could not calm myself with the favorable turn of fate. Doubt is the psychic region of unlimited possibilities.

Analysis led me back to the above-mentioned discussion which had occasioned my doubts. At the moment that Dora opposed my views and sided with my adversary, I felt a fleeting but violent impulse which can be expressed something like this: I hate her so much for this that I could choke her. The intensity of this feeling is explainable by my extreme jealousy which already made me interpret Dora's theoretical views as an indication of her tendency to be unfaithful. My obsessional act appears as self-punishment for my evil

* Later I was astonished at the absurdity of my thinking. In the second eventuality, if Dora were unfaithful and I were killed, I would hardly have time to recognize the result of my statement of the problem.

† Now this "chance," too, seems highly suspicious to me. Despite all the circumstances that favored my bumping into that man, it is quite probable that I unconsciously brought it about myself.

wish. Because I wanted to kill Dora, I am to be killed myself. In the substitution of my compulsive ideas, too, my death is linked with Dora's unfaithfulness; my death wish against her, after all, emerged in the face of the possibility that she could bestow her affections on someone else. It is permissible to ask at this point whether most self-made divine judgments of this type which are often found in compulsive neurotics do not prove to be psychic reactions to hostile wishes in the service of a tendency toward self-punishment.* On the basis of this insight, psychoanalysis would be able to provide a deeper understanding of many customs in the life of primitive peoples and of seemingly strange legal practices (e.g., medieval ordeals).

VEILED AND RATIONALIZED DEATH WISHES

Let us cite some examples of compulsive connections (fear, reflections, impulses, etc.) the analysis of which aims particularly at recognizing their multifarious disguises and primary motivations.

Psychoanalysis is well suited to interpreting a strange letter which I received at the time of Dora's illness. In those days I was giving German lessons to a foreigner, a young lady who was under psychoanalytic treatment for hysteria. From conversations with me she knew about my relationship with Dora, but she had never seen her or spoken with her. In view of this it struck me that after every lesson she inquired about Dora's condition with excessive interest. Since the woman wished to become familiar with German epistolary style, she was supposed to write me a letter. Some passages in this practice letter confirmed my supposition that her exaggerated solicitude about the well-being of a complete stranger like Dora permitted one to conclude that there was an unconscious hostile current in her. These passages go as follows: "Now I ask myself and you: How is Miss

---

* This view serves to elucidate the mechanism of a compulsive act in Arthur Schnitzler's play *Das weite Land*. Director Aigner has cheated on his wife; he has admitted it and the two have agreed to get a divorce. In discussing this with Friedrich Hofreiter, Aigner tells him in this connection about the dangerous first scaling of a mountain.

Aigner: Do you know when I first climbed the tower from which you have just returned? It was quite soon after I had separated from my wife.

Friedrich: Do you mean to say that there is some connection here?

Aigner: In a manner of speaking. . . . I am not saying that I was seeking death; I could have found death more easily than that. But at that time I didn't care about living. It may be that I was trying to invoke a divine judgment.

Dora? I regret that I have not asked you to phone me the latest news about her condition, because I am very worried. You will probably have to laugh at my letter, and perhaps there will also be some psychoanalytic explanations, right? Now I hear the rolling of carriages; they are coming from a wedding—poor people, unhappy celebration! . . . I hope you are spending this day well." As the lady told me the next day, she had on the previous day been uneasy and increasingly worried about Dora's illness. After overcoming her resistance, she herself was able to give an explanation of her very strange emotions. (*Cf.* the passage "perhaps there will also be some psychoanalytic explanations.") Her exaggerated solicitude was a psychic reaction to death wishes against Dora. She had unconsciously wished that I were still unattached and would want to marry her. Thus sexual envy was the reason for her enmity toward Dora. She hypocritically wished me a good day—that is, good news about Dora's state of health. This is a hypocritical wish because it conceals the opposite wish that aims at a hoped-for turn for the worse in Dora's condition. It seems striking that the preceding passage in the letter abruptly and without any apparent connection refers to some wedding. The very pessimistic view of this celebration does not harmonize with the other views and wishes. An unconscious factor was at work here: Associations that were in the service of her complexes and connected the sight of a wedding celebration that meant nothing to her with thoughts of my future marriage to Dora caused the wedding to be replaced in her mind by the gloomy image of a funeral procession. She wishes that Dora would die and not marry me.

Similar to this case, though much more complicated, is the case of two sisters who have the most affectionate feelings for each other. Viewed superficially, the solicitude of one sister about the other, as expressed in constant questions and warnings (Aren't you going to catch cold? Do you have a headache? Do you have palpitations?), was touching, but it was all the more striking because the two sisters, who were about the same age, were in excellent health. My analysis of a phobia-like trait in one of the sisters convinced me that evil, hostile currents lurked behind such extreme solicitude. For Erna, the younger sister, it was horrible when she had to be in a room in which another person was sleeping. She told me that the sleeping person seemed dead to her and that this filled her with fright. In the final stage of this phobia its substance changed to the point where Erna had the same feelings if she had to spend some time in a room with a person whose eyes were closed. She never felt afraid of dead persons; she spent long periods of time at the deathbeds of relatives without fear. But when she was alone with someone who was asleep (e.g., her mother), she felt like running away.

When there was some reason for her to stay in the room (illness, etc.), she tried to wake the sleeping person by making noise. Sometimes she managed to avoid compulsive acts through compassion. On such occasions she told herself: "The poor person has worked so hard all day or run so many errands; he (or she) must be tired, I must let him (or her) sleep." Analysis showed that this compassion was secondary in nature and a protective measure against her own impulses. I recapitulated the substance of her compulsive idea as told me by Erna; when I said, "So you feel like running away," Erna interrupted me: "Yes, at least that, or else like strangling the person in question." When I expressed my astonishment at such a surprising alternative, Erna explained that the reason for this latter impulse was her overwhelming anger at the sleeping person's failure to wake up. The reader will notice that this is an unsuccessful rationalization. "At the least run away" or "strangle" we shall interpret as one of the *hystera-protera* [inversions of the natural or logical order] so often observed in neurotics. The woman at first wants to strangle the person and then she wants to run away, because she is afraid of her own wish and its power that could be effected by the "omnipotence of thoughts." The example which Erna chose to explain her compulsive fear to me leaves no doubt that this fear related to a definite situation in her early childhood.*

Since early childhood the two sisters, Mary and Erna, have had the following strange custom: Mary is not allowed to fall asleep before Erna. This prescriptive right which Erna claims for herself is in force to this day, when both girls are in their middle twenties. This custom turns out to be a fine protective measure. Erna, the younger sister, once asked Mary to stay awake until she herself was asleep. The situation that constitutes the origin of Erna's compulsive

* "If it is possible to secure a specific example for one of the blurred generalizations of a compulsive neurosis, one may be certain that this example will be the original and real thing itself which was supposed to be concealed by the generalization." Freud, "Bemerkungen über einen Fall von Zwangsneurose," *Jahrbuch für psychoanalytische und psychopathologische Forschungen,* Vol. 3.

fear is as follows: When she was a child, Erna slept (as she still does) in the same room as her sister, who is one year older. One day, when she was watching her sleeping sister, Erna wished her sister would never wake up.* This feeling, which stemmed from a typical rivalry between children, conflicted with sisterly affection and the demands of the moral self; added to this was the expectation, already tinged with fear, that the evil wish would come true. Each time the sister was asleep, the memory of that repressed wish asserted itself as an anxiety which was regarded as groundless. The power of the wish and the belief in the "omnipotence of thoughts" were so great in Erna that she had to get relief through the above-mentioned protective measure. The wish that originally related to a definite person was later torn out of its special connection and, with the transferability peculiar to neurotic symptoms, extended to people generally in the form of a phobia. The generalization at the same time served to render the original occasion of the obsessional fear consciously inadequate and to extend the protection compulsion, the latter being typical of compulsive neurosis.

In Erna, too, the fear of death is present as a form of reaction to her death wishes directed against others. The most singular manifestation of this fear came when Erna was taking the baths at Bad Nauheim. When Erna was wrapped in blankets by an attendant after each carbonic bath and had to rest on a couch, she felt like a mummy, thought she was dead, and experienced all stages of fright. The unconscious idea of atonement found similar expression in another woman suffering from a compulsive neurosis. One day she felt "dead tired . . . as if all my limbs were paralyzed, quite beat," almost incapable of stirring. Analysis revealed that on the previous day she had desired to beat up a female friend who had offended her with some thoughtless words so that the friend might be in such a state. However, she had suppressed any indication of her rage and had even been especially charming toward her friend.

In later years Erna's death wish against her sister found expression in affect-free but obsessional reflections. One of the compulsive ideas that often emerged in her led her to reflect what her

---

* Inquiry revealed that when the sisters, who today are overly affectionate toward each other, were children, squabbles and bitter fights over dolls and the like were common occurrences.

life might have been like if she and not Mary had been the first-born. (This leads us to a more profound understanding of the biblical tale about Jacob and Esau.) Sometimes the conditional clause was changed: . . . if she had been the only child of her parents. In the latter form it came closer to the original formulation of the compulsive idea and its affective basis.

A point at which Erna's hostility toward Mary erupted was a surprising slip of the tongue. Mary had became engaged to a young man, but a short time later this man had bestowed his affections on another girl, so Mary had had to dissolve the engagement. Discussing this with a girl friend, Erna expressed her satisfaction at the fact that her sister had gotten over this first grave disappointment so quickly. She added: "After all, what good would it have done Mary to marry N.? In a year she would have been a widow." When her friend called her attention to this *lapsus linguae,* Erna was very surprised and explained she had meant to say that Mary would have been a divorcée.

In Mary the reaction to her hostility toward Erna took the hypocritical form of exaggerated solicitude about her health, good spirits, etc., as well as fear that she might be run over. Nor did she miss any opportunity of praising her sister extravagantly—in order to insulate herself against her unconscious hatred, as it were, and assure herself of her (reactively heightened) love. I used an incident which seemed suitable for explaining the real nature of these reactive phenomena to try to convince Mary as gently as possible that her extreme solicitude about Erna was traceable to repressed death wishes. Her answer is worth noting: "That's not true. I have plenty of suitors." Like psychoneurotic symptoms, this delightful rebuff—I had not said anything about the presence of a sexual rivalry—reveals as much as it seeks to conceal. The second sentence reveals the real primary reason for her unconsciously hostile attitude toward Erna: sexual envy. This and similar indirect confirmations can be compared with the words which the great benefactor on the Austrian throne is made to say in certain historical pulp novels: "You will never learn my name. I am Emperor Joseph."

Erna betrayed her death wish against Mary by her *lapsus linguae*. At this point I would like to mention briefly two cases which also belong to the psychopathology of everyday life and present themselves to psychoanalytic investigation as reactions to death wishes. A man mentioned to a friend that an aunt had informed him she had willed her house to him. The thoughts emerging in him were revealed by the following words: "But I don't know the apothecary status of the house." The man explained this phrase, a mixture of "hypothecary" and "apothecary,"* by saying that it was due to his having perceived, but not apperceived, the sign on the drugstore across the street. But the unconscious reason for this lapse was that the sight of the apothecary combined with the man's preconscious thoughts. In an apothecary one can buy poison. The slip of the tongue was a breakthrough of the man's wish, rejected by his conscious, to remove his aunt by poisoning her and thus gain possession of the prospective house at an earlier date.†

A woman could not remember the address of her fiancé although he had been living in the same apartment for a long time. When she wrote him, she felt tempted to put the address "Bognergasse" on the envelope. Analysis revealed that while walking on Bognergasse with her fiancé one day, she had had strong feelings of rage because her fiancé had voiced concern about her lack of thrift. Her anger at him must have been very intense, because it mounted to the point of a death wish which was immediately suppressed and regretted. The woman's fiancé actually lives on Bleichergasse.‡ The name of that street was repressed by the woman's memory of the death wish because it connoted something unpleasant. As Freud has pointed out, in dreams pallor is an unmistakable death symbol.§ The substitute name Bognergasse which came to mind was, among other associations, determined by the unconscious memory of the occasion of the death wish (scene on Bognergasse).

Such examples which prove the effect of unconscious death wishes could be multiplied at will. The persons in whose speech and action tendencies of this kind lead to symptomatic acts illustrate the reverse of Balaam in Jewish history: they want to bless and yet, under the compulsion of unconscious processes, they must curse.

---

* *Translator's note*: The words in the original are *apothekenfrei, Hypotheken,* and *Apotheken.*

† As a homeowner the man hoped to win the woman he loved.

‡ *Translator's note*: *Bleich* is the German word for "pale."

§ Cf. the interpretation of "paleness" in a version of Shakespeare's *Merchant of Venice* by Freud. ("Das Motiv der Kästchenwahl," *Imago,* 1913.)

A few cases of the unconscious continuation and secondary motivation of death wishes seem to me so illustrative of the general mechanism that I will not fail to adduce them here. The first case I owe to a young widow who related it to me as one of the strangest things that ever happened to her. During a serious illness of her seven-year-old son the wish that he might die arose in her, and of course she rejected it with horror. Later she explained this wish to herself by reasoning that afterwards (i.e., after his death) she would no longer have any ties to the life she hated and that she could then kill herself. She said the child was the only bond she still had to existence. I soon recognized that this motivation was a successful rationalization of repressed sexual desires and also that her disgust with life stemmed from a conflict which led to sexual rejection. Around that time she had been wooed by a young man whose courtship she would have liked to be successful. Certain family considerations, however, made a wedding appear out of the question. On the other hand, she felt strong moral inhibitions to giving herself to the young man without being his wife. One of the greatest obstacles to her desires was her small son, who, as she said, reminded her of her "dignity as a mother and a woman." The prospect of being condemned to sexual continence at such an early age was hardly a cheerful one. Added to this was her affection for the young man which was about to drive her to transcend all bounds of convention. The wish which emerged frequently during her son's illness was directed against the child as the obstacle to her sexual enjoyment. If the child died, she could follow her heart.*

A rather hidden method of effectuating death wishes is swearing by the lives of dear ones. I know a case in which a woman swore as follows: If I do such-and-such, may my husband die. She now had to keep reflecting whether she really had not done something and whether she had not taken a false oath; she was constantly under the spell of fear that (thanks to the "omnipotence of thoughts") her oath might lead to her husband's death. Since she could not abandon her inclination to swear by the life, or by the death, of her husband

* In Popper-Lynkeus's book *Phantasien eines Realisten* there is a story, "Im Postwagen," which contains a similar example of the power of the sexual drive. A woman who falls in love at first sight with a traveling companion pushes her small sleeping son from the moving mail carriage because he might interfere with sexual intercourse between the two.

and her anxiety mounted, she got some relief by limiting her oaths in this fashion: If this is not so, may my husband die this very day. This way her doubts and her anxiety were of just one day's duration. As she herself admitted, she was curious to know whether her oath had any consequences for the life of her husband. It is worth noting how close such oaths, being cast in the form of a conditional clause, come to the formulation of all compulsive ideas.

A man I know who is under psychoanalytic treatment for compulsive neurosis often has an impulse to throw his half-smoked cigarette into the courtyard of his apartment house where easily inflammable merchandise is stored. He frequently does so and is subsequently tortured by doubts whether he has not committed arson. He is then under the compulsion to stand by the window and look down into the courtyard until there no longer is reason to fear that a fire will break out. The fantasies which precede and follow this impulse explain its significance: The man imagines how the burning cigarette causes a fire that slowly spreads through the house; all efforts of the fire brigade to extinguish it are in vain and all inhabitants of the house are killed by the fire and the smoke. He can see these scenes with hallucinatory clarity and feels quite comfortable with these thoughts. Finally he tells himself (the good man thinks of himself last) that he is, after all, in the house himself and faces the same danger. He hears himself crying out for help in vain and sees himself lost beyond hope. The fantasy about the destruction of all is now followed, as atonement and self-punishment, by fear for his own life.

Another neurotic was also occupied in thought with his own death. He liked to fashion a daydream that proceeded from the question what he would do if a physician assured him that he would have to die within a certain period of time.* He imagined that then he would taste all the enjoyments which his neurosis now prevented him from having. He would spend money lavishly, have sexual intercourse as often as he could without fear of possible infection (he suffers from fear of infection and bacteria), etc. To understand this fantasy correctly, it has to be read backwards, somewhat like Hebrew writing. This neurotic's father once forbade him to masturbate, and

* This case can also serve as an interesting example of the neurotic attitude toward time.

this prohibition trauma had such a strong aftereffect that the patient regarded his father as an obstacle to every enjoyment. The death wish that arose against the disturber was followed and expiated by fears regarding the danger to his own life. Because as a child he often asked himself how much longer his father was going to live, he now fears that a doctor would predict only a very short lifespan for him. (Self-punishment.) We deem it probable that the doctor constitutes a father substitute. (Thus the death sentence threatens to come from the father himself.)

But since he has to die, he and his father are quits and he can afford all enjoyments. Here the neurotic symptom, like a "biographical dream," comes close to the presentation of a developmental impediment in that it constitutes a *hysteron proteron*: the patient was disturbed in his infantile sexual activity by his father and therefore directed a death wish against him; he atones for this wish by the prospect of his own death. His daydream shows not only this self-punishment but also the origin of the death wishes in the eruption of the repressed feelings. The reconstructed scheme of the sequence of wish and punishment, or fear of punishment, can be illustrated by a little point which he told me about. When he is at a party, he sometimes says to himself: "I'm having a good time; I'm doing all right." Then it immediately seems to him as though some other voice inside him were saying to him: "Just wait, fellow, I'll show you that you are just imagining your good mood and that you really aren't doing all right." He told me that invariably something bad happens to him the same evening—something goes wrong, he loses an illusion, etc.

The same compulsive neurotic also indicated in a rather blunt way that he harbors such bad wishes against me as well. His parents used to have a small dog that they loved. This dog came down with croup, and the patient declared that the dog would have to be sent away because he was afraid of being infected. The worried parents, ready to fulfill their ill son's every desire, deliberated on what was to be done with the beloved animal. The patient counseled them: "Why don't you give him to Dr. Reik!" It does not matter to psychoanalytic investigation whether I could have become dangerously infected. The decisive thing is that the patient believed the presence of the dog to be a danger to life and wanted me to be exposed to this danger. But consciously he only wanted to make me a present. It should be added that this compulsive neurotic with great pleasure (or, as he puts it, with sadistic delight) forces other persons to touch those objects which are "impossible" (taboo) for him and whose touch he dreads like death itself.

If we survey the numerous cases of an unconscious aftereffect of death wishes which have passed in review before us, we recognize its derivation from drives by inferring the cause from the effect. In the psychogenesis of death wishes, repressed sexual feelings play the main part; however, they are usually welded together with marked elements of the ego drive. This intertwining and enfolding of drives is made possible by the narcissistic attitude which is also the origin of the belief in the "omnipotence of thoughts." It may be surmised that in persons who have such violent wishes against their dearest ones the sadistic component is especially strongly developed constitutionally.

One compulsive neurotic gave me the following description: "When another person is even slightly annoyed by a fellow human being, there immediately arises in me this wish for the latter: Drop dead!"

The force and the intensity of the emotions of such persons are a constant source of astonishment to us, as is hatred as the constant companion of love.

The enormous incidence of death wishes in drives and affects may be frightening, but no unbiased observer will be able to deny it. The reproach that these sexual and hostile wishes were suggested to the patients by psychoanalysis seems absurd. Human nature was not fashioned by *us*.

If this reproach makes any sense at all, it must be leveled at a higher authority. When God viewed the world on the sixth day of Creation, he saw that it was good. Perhaps we shall do well to add to the anthropomorphic image of God which we have fashioned for ourselves the fine virtue of modesty.

The Psychoanalytic Review
Vol. 65, No. 1, 1978

REIK, SCHNITZLER, FREUD, AND "THE MURDERER": The Limits of Insight in Psychoanalysis*

Murray H. Sherman†

"Do you remember the novel *The Murderer* by Schnitzler?" This was the surprising question that Sigmund Freud addressed to Theodor Reik during a psychoanalytic session.[1] Reik attributes an almost magically curative effect to this question and to his own amazed and insightful response. There is a long and complex history surrounding this incident, the understanding of which may illuminate not only the relationships between Reik, Schnitzler, and Freud but also the determining role that literature played in Reik's life.

Freud's question and the life situation in which it was embedded are viewed here as a kind of nodal point in time that caught Reik sharply in its focus. What kind of insight did Reik derive from *The Murderer* and upon what factors was this insight based. Some psychoanalytic interpretation of this work is offered and certain aspects of the relationship between Reik, Schnitzler, and Freud are described. However, the major emphasis is upon the relationship between Reik's own life behavior and the nature of his insight.

---

* Reprinted with minor changes and with permission of the publisher, from *Modern Austrian Literature,* Vol. 10, Nos. 3-4, 1977, pp. 195-216.

† I am deeply indebted to Jeffrey B. Berlin for bringing Reik's correspondence with Schnitzler to my attention, for his valuable translations of this material, and for unlimited assistance with related literature and suggestions for this essay. Roy Huss has been most generous and helpful with his cogent suggestions and editorial assistance. I thank Arthur Reik for his kind permission to publish excerpts from his father's letters and other documentation. My sincere thanks to Miriam Reik for her insightful comments, which have been incorporated in this article. Heinrich Schnitzler has kindly made available portions of his father's unpublished diaries.

0033-2836/78/1300-0068 $00.95 © 1978 N.P.A.P.

Reik himself has supplied a good deal of the story behind Freud's question about *The Murderer*[2] in *Fragment of a Great Confession* (1949). However, as Reik explicitly states in *Fragment*, and as is implied by the title, he provides only a part of the story. Discretion to others, as well as to himself, led Reik to withhold certain data, but this fact is less significant than Reik's total relationship to literature and to the literary figures who loomed as giants in his own life history.[3]

Reik knew Schnitzler personally from his early days in Vienna. The correspondence between these two men, recently brought to light and published by Bernd Urban[4] and by Jeffrey B. Berlin,[5] permits us to date certain events, as well as understand the character of their relationship. In addition, some of Schnitzler's feelings toward Reik and psychoanalysis, as described by Schnitzler in his as yet unpublished diaries, have become available through the kindness of Heinrich Schnitzler and also Bernd Urban.[6]

The first entry[7] regarding Schnitzler's interest in Reik is a brief note in Schnitzler's diary dated March 5, 1912, in which he responds favorably to having read Reik's recently published study on Beer-Hofmann.[8] On June 27, 1912, Schnitzler refers to "a not uninteresting study" that Reik had just published. This was "Arthur Schnitzler vor dem 'Anatol': Psychoanalytisches,"[9] which appeared in the issue of *Pan* having the same publication date as Schnitzler's June entry. Reik had noted the psychological fascination of Schnitzler's work, compared him to Heine, and took particular note of Schnitzler's theme of fantasy versus reality. Schnitzler's reaction was a positive one, but even at this earliest contact with Reik and before meeting him, he voiced his reservations about psychoanalysis; the diary entry continues: "Only toward the end does it [Reik's article] run into the fixed psychoanaytic ideas." By "fixed ideas" Schnitzler was referring to the predominant analytic focus upon the Oedipus complex.

It was at this time that Reik first wrote to Schnitzler, sent him samples of his writing, and asked to meet him. Nothing could have made Reik more ecstatic than the response he received, as we observe in the opening sentence of Reik's first available letter of July 2, 1912, to Schnitzler: "Your so very gracious note has embellished a summer evening that threatened to become quite melancholy, with a deeply and sincerely felt joy."[10] Reik was twenty-four at this time, Schnitzler had passed his fiftieth birthday, and the adulation reflected in these lines continues through much of the correspondence. Schnitzler became one of the major figures in Reik's life, one whom he emulated both in his written work and in his actual life.

Reik's father had died in 1906, and his mother in 1910. It was in this same year that he met Sigmund Freud, who became by far the most predominant person in his life. It was also during this same interval, in March 1912, that Reik first wrote to Richard Beer-Hofmann[11]* and established a relationship that was rather comparable to that with Schnitzler. These three men—Freud, Schnitzler, and Beer-Hofmann—replaced the parents whom Reik had recently lost. Reik himself wrote a great deal about the death of his father,[12] and throughout his life he continued to be much preoccupied with the theme of love and death—a topic that dominates much of Schnitzler's work.

A few words about Theodor Reik may help describe his position in the world of psychoanalysis and literature. Born on May 12, 1888, Reik grew up in Vienna at a time when Freud and Schnitzler were being both acclaimed and pilloried in that city.[13] One can readily see how these controversial figures would have appealed to a youth drawn toward intellectual rebelliousness, as most creative writers are.

Reik became an integral member of the dedicated group of analysts around Freud, and he contributed significantly to analytic literature from 1911 on.[14] Reik practiced psychoanalysis in Vienna, and later in Berlin, and moved to the Hague in 1934 after fleeing from the Nazis. He came to the United States in 1938 and lived and practiced in New York City until his death on December 31, 1969.

Reik's earliest contributions established him as one of the few masters of applied psychoanalysis (that is, psychoanalysis used to study culture, literature, and art) along with Hanns Sach (1881-1947) and Otto Rank (1883-1939), both of whom had preceded him in the Vienna Psychoanalytic Society by a few years. Reik succeeded Rank as Secretary of the Society in 1918 and remained in this post until 1928.

Reik first became acquainted with Freud's name in 1910, while he was studying psychology at the University of Vienna. Reik's

* Richard Beer-Hofmann (1866-1945), Austrian dramatist and writer.

psychology professor had made disparaging remarks in class about *The Interpretation of Dreams*, but Reik's own response to the book was enthusiastic and marked the start of a lifetime of devotion to psychoanalysis. He began attending Freud's lectures at the University, wrote to him, and was cordially received. Reik's earliest major work, *Ritual: Psychoanalytic Studies* (1919),[15] was awarded a *prix d'honneur* for the outstanding contribution to applied psychoanalysis and led Freud to call Reik "one of our best hopes."[16]

Reik, who was well grounded in literature long before he came to psychology and psychoanalysis, named his first child Arthur, after Schnitzler,[17] reflecting his intense admiration of this literary giant.

In the unhappy home of his childhood, young Theodor turned to books as an escape from the tragic atmosphere around him. His mother was a mournful and grief-stricken woman who had lost her own mother at so early an age that she had no memory of her. She often mentioned this to her children and then commented on their own better fortune in this regard. Mrs. Reik had also lost four of six children by the time Theodor was born. He lived in a household where death was a hovering presence. Reik's habit of reading while eating his meals drove his mother to distraction. Reik's immersion in literature was, in fact, one of his most outstanding characteristics and directly related to a rich and deep fantasy life that sustained him. Although his doctorate was awarded in psychology, the largest number of courses listed on his transcript were in French and German literature, and the topic of his dissertation was *Flaubert and His "Temptation of St. Anthony": A Contribution to the Psychology of Artists* (1912).[18] Even at this early date psychology revealed itself to Reik as a form of literature. Schnitzler was to be most instrumental in reinforcing this feeling.

Until as late as December 1918, Reik was actually undecided as to his career in psychoanalysis. In Reik's letter to Schnitzler of December 11, 1918, he states that he has been "successful in finding a position as political editor of the Vienna *Zeit*." To those who are acquainted with Reik's almost total indifference to politics in his later years, this fact might seem amazing. However, in the years following his father's death in 1906 and until about 1919, Reik was actually quite desperate about how he would make a living and simply survive. He generally sought editorial positions of various kinds, relying upon his writing ability and excellent command of language and literature, but at one time Reik applied to Max Reinhardt, the prominent theatrical director, for any sort of job that might be available in his production group.[19]

The correspondence between Reik and Schnitzler graphically portrays Reik's growth from an anxious and insecure youth who was quite importunate in besieging Schnitzler with requests for help in finding work, to the mature and self-reliant psychoanalyst, who had himself achieved a measure of international renown. Reik's earlier insecurity is portrayed quite dramatically in his letter to Schnitzler dated January 4, 1914:

> This Bohemian kind of life that has been forced on me torments me as much as does the miserable financial condition in which I find myself as a consequence. I would be eternally grateful to you, my dear Herr Doctor, if you would put in a good word for me with one of your influential friends. Of course, I would prefer a position as an editor, a dramatic advisor, or a secretary, but I would also agree to any other type of work, as long as I could make a living from it.

The later phases of the correspondence refer to exchanges of publications between the two men, arrangements for visits, and comments by Reik about how he still made use of Schnitzler's writing in his own work. In a letter of November 17, 1929, Reik writes,

> In a few weeks I will take the liberty of sending you a new book about Goethe [*Why Did Goethe Leave Friederike?*][20] in which your story "The Fate of the Baron von Leisenbohg" plays a special part. You will recognize from this how much your books are in my thoughts even now.

Schnitzler himself was friendly but more impersonal and aloof with Reik. He respected Reik's work but did not respond in close terms to him. Reik's correspondence with Beer-Hofmann conveys a warmer tone. In each of these relationships Reik was looking up to a man who, he felt, towered above him.

In 1912 Schnitzler and Reik sat together and analyzed the dream of one of Schnitzler's literary figures (Georg of *The Road into the Open*). In 1921 Reik referred one of his patients to Schnitzler for consultation.* Their relationship thus encompassed a certain de-

---

* See B. Urban, this issue, p. 147.

gree of collaboration. However, Reik's feelings toward Schnitzler were those of deep admiration and devotion. Schnitzler's attitude toward Reik was ambivalent and perhaps condescending or even somewhat disdainful.

Schnitzler's earliest contact with Freud went back to 1886, when he attended and reported upon a meeting at which Freud spoke on the subject of male hysteria,[21] and in 1888 he wrote a book review in which he took Freud's part in the controversy over the medical use of cocaine.[22] Schnitzler also reviewed Freud's early translation of Charcot's *Leçons du Mardi.*[23] Freud's admiration for *Paracelsus* and other Schnitzler works is now well known,[24] and Jones states that Freud and Schnitzler knew each other personally.[25] However, it is certainly strange that these two men, thinking so similarly about the relationship of sexual response to personal destiny, delayed meeting each other in person for many years.[26]

Schnitzler was probably intrigued by Freud's libido theory, his concept of the unconscious, and later with Freud's theory of the death instinct and repetition compulsion. He did not, however, accept Freud's concepts of infantile sexuality and incest wishes.[27] Further, Schnitzler became annoyed when analysts read unconscious motives that he had not intended into his characters. His response here was not unlike that of most people who do not like to be told what they think when they do not think that they think it! Schnitzler responded in his diary by characterizing psychoanalysis as having "fixed ideas," being "one-sided," or even "monomaniacal."[28]

To a certain extent, Reik represented to Schnitzler an ambassador or symbol of psychoanalysis, conceivably a kind of "stand-in" for Freud, and this enabled him to express his feelings about Freud and psychoanalysis more easily than he otherwise did. A psychoanalyst might term this a form of displacement. At any rate, Schnitzler's mixed feelings toward Reik are reflected in his diary entry for December 8, 1923: "[Reik] is an intelligent man [*kluger mensch*], very erudite, and like all psychoanaysts, somewhat monomaniacal."

Reik's most striking encounter with Schnitzler was not a real one but occurred in one of Schnitzler's dreams, which was recorded in his diary for July 7, 1913:

> Now I am somewhere with Dr. Reik. He becomes wittily intimate which I angrily refuse, even pushing him away. When he became

> offended, I was sorry and I immediately tried to be good to him. A more learned person is there (Dr. [Hanns] Sachs?, invisible). I speak up, "The next great man will be the one who assigns psychoanalysis its exact boundaries," which to my astonishment Reik agrees with. . . . Interpretations: . . . The intimacy of Reik, characteristic of psychoanalysts who search out intimate details. The more learned Dr. Sachs. . . . My criticism of psychoanalysis does not need more interpretation. . . . Agreement of Reik: The psychoanalyst [Alfred R. F.] Winterstein replied when I said "I do not agree with everything in your papers," "Neither do I."

It is interesting to note here that Schnitzler associates to his dream in much the same way as do patients and also analysts in standard psychoanalytic procedures. The dream itself illustrates an ambivalent attitude toward psychoanalysis and its representatives. Schnitzler may also have inwardly sensed the same *Doppelgänger* effect (the fear of encountering one's double),[29] as Freud acknowledged in his famous letter of May 14, 1922, to Schnitzler,[30] and he may have been intrigued and also vaguely repelled by this feeling on much the same basis as Freud.

Among those writers whose influence Reik specifically mentions are Dostoevsky, Nietzsche, Hauptmann, Schiller, Grillparzer, Nestroy, and especially Goethe, Shakespeare, France, Heine, Flaubert, and Beer-Hofmann. Goethe's statement that all his writings could simply be regarded as "fragments of a great confession," provided, of course, the title of Reik's own *Fragment* (and may also have influenced the title of Freud's "Fragment of an Analysis of a Case of Hysteria"). Reik himself describes the influence of Goethe's writing in *Fragment* at some length.[31] He also speaks of the influence of Heine,[32] and his mode of identification with this poet may be surmised from the remark in *Listening with the Third Ear* that he sometimes regards psychoanalysis as "less a profession than a calamity!"[33] Does this not recall Heine's comment that Judaism often seems "less a religion than a misfortune"? Reik's abundant use of wit, subtlety, irony, and nuance may have been much influenced also by the writing of Anatole France.[34]

However, for general themes and style of writing no writer exerted more influence on Reik than Schnitzler. The motifs of love and death and especially of the omnipresence of death resound throughout all of Reik's work. At the very first meeting of the Vienna Psychoanalytic Society that Reik attended, on November

15, 1911, he presented an essay entitled "On Death and Sexuality," and the writers whose work he mentioned were Flaubert, Beer-Hofmann—and Schnitzler.[35]

Schnitzler's "The Fate of the Baron von Leisenbohg"[36] impressed itself deeply on Reik's mind and later led to his article "The 'Omnipotence of Thought' in Arthur Schnitzler" (1913).[37] The plot of this narrative centers upon a Baron who learns of a curse invoked by the dying lover of a young woman whom the Baron himself had long been courting. The curse pronounced instant death on the first man to make love to the woman after the lover's own death. When the Baron discovers that the woman has treacherously given herself to him in order to discharge the curse so that she can then turn to another man, he suddenly falls dead. To Reik, this story illustrated Schnitzler's understanding of how thoughts could kill.

In a much later publication, *The Need To Be Loved* (1963),[38] Reik uses Schnitzler's "Redegonda's Diary"[39] to illustrate one aspect of erotomania, the illusion of being pursued in love by another person. This story tells of a young lawyer who indulges in detailed erotic fantasies about a young married woman to whom he does not dare speak. His fantasies progress to the point where he becomes her lover and they run away together. Suddenly, the young woman's husband informs the lawyer that his wife has died, and when upon reading her diary he discovers that she had reciprocated the lawyer's fantasies, the husband challenges him to a duel and kills him. Again, Reik was struck by how fantasies could lead to death, especially in a love relationship.

In addition to the well-known *Arthur Schnitzler as Psychologist,*[40] Reik wrote "The Relations of the Sexes in Schnitzler" (1913),[41] and he reviewed *Frau Beate and Her Son* in 1914.[42] After Schnitzler's death in 1931, Reik produced a memorial article with the paradigmatic title of "Death and Love: In Memory of Arthur Schnitzler."[43] Reik also devotes a chapter of *The Secret Self* (1952) to *Hands Around.*[44]

Other writings of Schnitzler to which Reik refers include *The Road into the Open,*[45] *Intermezzo,*[46] *The Big Wurstel Puppet Theater,*[47] *The Wide Country,*[48] *The Last Mask,*[49] *The Lonely Road,*[50] and *The Call of Life.*[51] There was no other contemporary writer to whom Reik alluded so often.[52] The theme in Schnitzler's writing that impressed Reik far beyond any other was the close connection between love and death, and particularly the demonic influence of thoughts and fantasies in causing the death of someone in love. These influences were felt many years before Freud's question regarding *The Murderer*.

One other important element in Schnitzler's writing that impressed Reik was that of the sudden surprise endings in the stories as well as in his plays,[53] and it is of interest that one of the few American writers to whom Reik alluded was O. Henry.[54] Reik indicates the crucial significance of surprise in his analysis of the psychology of wit,[55] and he often alludes to surprise in dissecting the unconscious communication between patient and psychoanalyst. In this connection, one may note that the title of Reik's major work on technique is *Surprise and the Psychoanalyst* (1935),[56] which was later incorporated into *Listening with the Third Ear* (1948).

The general form that Reik's writing took was also significantly influenced by the feuilleton, (i.e., cultural journalism), which was so prevalent in the era in which he grew up. Reik well recognized this influence and tried to avoid it. In a letter to Schnitzler of December 20, 1913, he wrote, "I strove with immense effort to transcend the usual feuilletonistic way of thinking." However, just six months later, June 20, 1914, he wrote that he "would prefer [a position in] the feuilleton section and theater criticism." Reik was sometimes torn between the objectivity of science and the emotional appeal of literary effects, but in his most personal and characteristic writing literature easily won out.

Schnitzler's own acknowledged response to Reik is best summarized in a letter dated April 2, 1914, that he wrote to Hans Henning in defense of Reik's *Arthur Schnitzler as Psychologist*:

> It is understandable that I do not like to discuss writings that concern me. This time it is all the more difficult because I know Dr. Reik personally, hold him in high esteem, and, furthermore, have made no secret of the fact, either before or after the publication of his book, that I have scruples about the onesidedness of the psychoanalytic method practiced by him and other students of Freud, regardless of the very interesting and sometimes even correct results it may lead to. Then, too, because I have been asked to express an opinion to you, a man who has the intention of writing about the Reik book himself and in this connection, like it or not, about me as well. I would therefore prefer to limit my remarks from an author's point of view to those aspects of Theodor Reik's presenta-

> tion which seem to me likeable and valuable in a larger context: Reik draws attention to something that certain professional critics usually ignore: namely, my depiction of non-erotic human relationships as between siblings, parents and children, and friends. He also points out various deeper psychological connections, though he does not exactly say the last word about them and in some cases probably is not absolutely correct. In addition: from conversations with Reik (no more than two or three thus far) I have gained the conviction (though he still has not) that in the future he will look upon Freud's methods of interpretation (regardless of the depth of knowledge of human nature from which the basic ideas might originally have emerged) not as the sole and only path to salvation, but as one among many that leads to the secret of poetic creation, at times, however, into vagueness or error. Surely you will be kind enough to send me your critique when it is available. For now, let me thank you most cordially for your kind interest.[57]

To a psychoanalyst Arthur Schnitzler warrants attention on many counts. His writings parallel those of Freud in their early focus upon the psychological significance of sexual behavior, and as has been demonstrated many times, his works may be used to illustrate such psychoanalytic concepts, for example, as Oedipal attachments (in *Frau Beate and Her Son*),[58] the omnipotence of thought (in *The Fate of the Baron . . .*),[59] and the significance of transitional objects (also in *The Fate of the Baron . . .*).[60] In addition, Schnitzler's characters bear such uncanny likeness to real persons that their emotional reactions, thought processes, and behavior may be actually diagnosed or even in a sense "psychoanalyzed." In this regard, Robert O. Weiss has convincingly demonstrated the various symptoms of hysteria, hypochondriasis, ambivalence, paranoid delusions, and others, all in the character of Robert in *Flight into Darkness*.[61] Reik himself epitomizes the psychoanalytic understanding of Schnitzler's plots and characters.

To psychologists and sociologists and others concerned with the concept of role and role-playing, Schnitzler's characters also hold particular appeal. Reinhard Urbach, a literary critic, has indicated how Schnitzler's deep awareness of various role behaviors penetrate into the deepest meanings of life itself:

> Role-playing became the life style of society, not as a theatrical, pathetic, or affectatious exhibition, not as a play before God, but as a game of individuals with each other, everywhere and constantly.

> In the world of role-playing there are no barriers of class, birth, or wealth. Anyone who wishes may play. Power goes to the most accomplished player. The society of players claims unlimited pleasure in all areas of life, particularly in the erotic.[62]

Since our main focus will now be on *The Murderer,* a brief statement of its plot will be given, followed by some exploration of its psychoanalytic significance. The central character of *The Murderer* is a young man, Alfred, who goes on a long ocean voyage with his mistress, Elise, while still in love with a wealthy young woman, Adele, whom he hopes to marry upon his return. Elise has informed Alfred of a heart ailment before the voyage, but her illness worsens during the trip. Alfred has also been warned by the ship's physician that sex is dangerous to Elise's precarious health, and although Elise knows this, she prefers to continue their lovemaking and to die in Alfred's arms rather than to abstain. However, Alfred is impatient for Elise's death so that he can marry Adele, and he poisons Elise and makes it appear that the cause of her death has been sexual excitement. Alfred then returns home unsuspected, but upon his return discovers that Adele is now planning to marry another man. She dismisses Alfred quite contemptuously, and he then allows himself to be killed in a duel.

Psychoanalytically, this plot epitomizes the split between the tender and aggressive aspects of sex. Tender feelings are directed toward one individual and the aggression felt in this relationship becomes directed toward someone else. A "normal" individual is able to combine these opposing feelings reasonably well in a meaningful and continuing relationship with another person. The emotionally disturbed individual may be driven, for example, to construct external obstacles to his own fulfillment toward which he can then direct his aggression while maintaining the relationship of tenderness. Freud has described this paradox:

> It can easily be shown that the psychical value of erotic needs is reduced as soon as their satisfaction becomes easy. An obstacle is required in order to heighten libido; and where natural resistances to satisfaction have not been sufficient men have at all times erected conventional ones so as to be able to enjoy love.[63]

In Alfred's case, he is able to love Elise when he first meets her. However, after he persuades Elise to give up her position as a correspondence clerk and she then devotes herself tenderly to him, the obstacle (of employment) has disappeared and he must then erect another. The obstacle eventually takes the form of an attachment to the unobtainable Adele, and in fact as soon as Alfred becomes fixated on Adele, Elise herself becomes the obstacle to fulfillment that must be eliminated. As the plot develops, Alfred's tender feelings toward Adele culminate in a determination to marry her, and the aggression toward Elise, who has now become the frustrating object, mounts until he murders her.

The Murderer contains a number of other illustrations of using obstacles to fulfillment in order to "be able to enjoy love." Elise's illness may be seen as an ultimate obstacle to her own fulfillment. The ocean voyage becomes an obstacle to Alfred, separating him from Adele. After Alfred returns to Adele, presumably free of obstacles, he finds another in the form of her engagement to marry another man. All these obstacles serve to frustrate the characters' emotional fulfillment by splitting their longings into differences that cannot become reconciled.

Freud's original statement of this split in feeling was described by him as one between "the *affectionate* and the *sensual* current."[64] However, he later recognized the primary significance of aggression and then theorized two major groups of instincts: love or libido (Eros), and death (Thanatos).[65] Aggression is derived from the death instinct (the individual's drive toward his own death), which becomes directed outward toward others. In actual life behavior Eros and Thanatos are always combined, or fused, but in pathological instances they may become separated, or defused. In Alfred's case we find an extreme defusion that eventuates in a literal acting out of the death instinct. At the end of the tale, Alfred's own death in a duel, which he seems deliberately to seek out, would be attributed by an analyst to unconscious guilt feelings stemming from his murder of Elise, as well as to the death instinct turned back upon the original source, the self.

From a psychological viewpoint, one criticism that could be directed at this story is that there is a discrepancy between Alfred's character and his actions. Alfred is portrayed as a weak and vain man, one prone to vacillate and to exploit women—hardly the man to coldly murder his sweetheart and walk away without a qualm. The theme of murder appears almost superimposed upon the character rather than growing out of his own emotions and drives.

There is a good deal more that could be described regarding the relationship of Schnitzler, Freud, and Reik to each other vis-à-vis psychoanalysis and literature, but the purpose here is to focus more narrowly on Reik's quite astounding reaction to Freud's question during an analytic session: "Do you remember the novel *The Murderer* by Schnitzler?" The entire schema of *Fragment* (1949), which is a kind of autobiographical confession, centers upon this question.

Reik begins the book with the sudden death of his father from a heart attack in 1906. Reik had been sent to the drug store for medicine to relieve his father's labored breathing. He ran as quickly as possible, but by the time he returned his father was dead.[66] Reik was seized by fits of remorse and anxiety and also, unaccountably, by sexual excitement. As if to atone for a crime, he suddenly felt compelled to read every last word that Goethe had ever written or that was written about Goethe. He spent whole days in the library reading his way through the complete works of Goethe and would travel miles on foot to view even an insignificant piece of paper on which Goethe had written a few words. The compulsion gradually abated over the course of the following year, and by this time Reik was a student in the University of Vienna.

Reik next recalls how, in 1929, he had published the monography *Why Did Goethe Leave Friederike?*[67] This work then follows almost in its entirety in *Fragment,* and Reik explains how the Goethe monograph had been influenced—at the time unconsciously—by his much earlier courtship and marriage to his first wife, Ella. He then recounts the story of this relationship.

Young Theodor first met Ella, who was two years younger than he, when they were children and Ella's family occupied the flat below the Reiks. Although they passed each other in the hallway, Reik was too shy to speak but merely showed off when he thought Ella was looking. When Reik was twelve, Ella's family moved away and he did not meet her again until age nineteen. At this time, he initiated a courtship of seven years which was burdened by the inordinate jealousy of Ella's father, who would not permit any suitors. Reik's visits had to remain secret, he could see her for only a half-hour, and he did not set foot in the household. Only when Ella's father was away on business could the two be together for a longer period of time. On these rare occasions, Theodor and Ella made excursions into the mountains and visited rural inns where they could lunch and dance.

Sometimes the two lovers quarreled about their favorite writers and composers. Reik told Ella about Goethe's romance with Friederike, Ella mentioned Richard Strauss, and Reik said he did not like Strauss but preferred Mahler. Ella repeated some gossip about Mahler and the two argued, then kissed and made up. After recounting these experiences Reik draws a parallel between the sexual conflict behind quarrels like these and the conflict felt by Goethe in his Friederike romance. In both cases there was a sexual conflict centering first upon the theme of love and then upon abandonment. Reik says that when he first read Goethe's story, he determined that he would never leave a beloved the way Goethe abandoned Friederike.

Reik resumes the narrative. After the quarrel, the two lovers went to an inn and danced to a waltz. It was at this time that Reik first encountered Ella's physical weakness and illness. She could not finish the waltz, gasped for breath, and was forced to sit down. Ella soon recovered, and Reik then recalled that he had been told that Ella had rheumatic fever and should not exert herself. After they parted that day, Reik grew melancholy, preoccupied with the evanescence of life and the certainty of death.

Reik suddenly interrupts his courtship story to tell of his concurrent sexual relationship with Vilma, twelve years older than he and a woman of far looser morals than Ella. He explains his reluctance and inhibitions with Ella and also mentions the urgency and undeniableness of his sexual drive.

In 1914 Theodor Reik and Ella Oratsch married. At the time Reik was living in Berlin, where he had been sent by Freud for an analysis with Karl Abraham. Although he was drafted into the Austrian army medical corps in 1915, he managed to be home for the birth of his son later that year. Reik served in the cavalry, was decorated for bravery in action, and was discharged in November 1918.[68]

After the war Reik became a prominent analyst in Vienna and developed a prosperous and productive career. However, the symptoms of rheumatic heart disease which Reik had first noted in Ella during the courtship soon developed into a chronic cardiac inflammation complicated by kidney infection. Reik says that constant invalidism turned his wife into an irritable, demanding woman, and he was forced into virtual slavery to support both her medical treatment and also her whims and expensive tastes.[69] He further says that he was forced to turn to other women for sexual satisfaction in order to "spare" his wife, and he speaks of several affairs, one of them dating to his service in Montenegro during the war and another with a nurse in the hospital where Ella was being treated.

Although Ella's physician had directly told Reik that sex was not dangerous to his wife, he writes,

> How could I disavow the visible signs of the bad influence it had on her? . . . It was as if Ella had unconsciously sensed my fear, because she seemed in a subtle way to encourage my lovemaking, but I am sure this was only under the impression that sexual satisfaction was a necessity for a man.[70]

Reik went to Freud for psychoanalytic therapy during the summer of 1935, while Freud was vacationing at Aussee in Austria. Reik had been suffering from neurotic anxiety symptoms since 1929, the same year he had published the Goethe study. He experienced heart palpitations that brought on fears of imminent death and had frequent attacks of dizziness, vomiting, and diarrhoea.[71] Reik also mentions that he had been seeing a young woman and that this relationship was becoming a serious one. "I had made the acquaintance of a girl who, many years younger than myself, attracted me in many ways, not only sexually."[72] In a later volume Reik identifies the young woman as Maria, his second wife.[73] One gathers that the relationship with Maria may well have inspired the writing of the Goethe monograph, and perhaps also have been the basic factor in the conflict underlying Reik's symptoms.

Freud made two comments in particular that produced a vivid impression on Reik. At the end of a session Freud said to Reik, "I would have thought you stronger."[74] Earlier in the same session had come Freud's question about *The Murderer*.

In applying that question to himself, Reik says that only then did he recognize that he had unconscious death wishes toward Ella, had unconsciously wished her dead so that he could marry Maria.

> I confessed [to Freud] that the thought had sometimes occurred to me to get a divorce from my wife, and to marry this girl, but I added that I knew, of course, that this was impossible: you cannot divorce a wife who is dangerously ill.[75]

Reik says that Freud's question was intended to give him insight into his unconscious death wishes toward Ella and that Freud's comment about thinking Reik stronger meant that he should have been strong enough to demonstrate moral courage in facing these unconscious death wishes.[76] However, Reik's interpretation of Freud's remark may have been only partly correct, and in this present essay further meanings that Freud may have intended are explored. The examination is based on (1) certain details in *The Murderer,* (2) a close examination of Reik's own comments in *Fragment,* (3) details from Reik's other publications, and (4) factual information made available to this writer.

Reik had been literally obsessed with fears of causing Ella's death as long before as 1913, when he anonymously published an article entitled "On the Effects of Unconscious Death Wishes."[77]* He discusses this article in *Fragment,* but gives only a partial review of its contents and omits the part that explicitly interprets his unconscious death wishes toward Ella *at that time.* The article describes an obsession that impressed itself on Reik's mind while he was courting Ella: "If I do not walk now to my sister in K., Dora [pseudonym for Ella] will die." Under the influence of this mysterious command, Reik did then walk to see his sister.[78]

The visit to his sister was related to lighting a *jahrzeit* candle to honor the anniversary of his father's death, and the unconscious thought behind the obsession was discovered by Reik to be, "If I do not go to Weidling and if I do not light the candle, Ella will die." In *Fragment* Reik states that the fear of causing Ella's death was derived from an unconscious death wish toward his father,[79] but in the original article Reik had additionally stated that the "death wish that lurks behind my obsessional idea is directed against [Ella]."[80] In the interval of thirty-six years between the article and *Fragment* Reik had pushed this original insight into his death wish toward Ella out of awareness, and he succeeded in avoiding it even in recounting the article itself.

Another aspect of the 1913 article casts light upon Reik's obsessions about death. In that article he speaks of the landlady's daughter Daisy, who interrupted Reik's work by coming into his room in the evening to chat. At that time he developed the obsession, "If I chat with Miss Daisy today, Dora [Ella] will die" (p. 55). Daisy may be

* See this Special Issue, pp. 55, 58.

a disguise or displacement for Reik's liaison with Vilma, and his obsessional thought would then have had the meaning, "If I have sexual relations with Vilma this evening, Ella will die." This may have been the actual origin or Reik's "unconscious death wishes" toward Ella, which grew from his overwhelming need to separate sex from love.

Also in 1913 Reik had written his article about Schnitzler's story "The Fate of the Baron von Leisenbohg,"[81] in which he stressed the magical power of thoughts that could kill. There was a close connection between what Reik read in Schnitzler, what actually transpired in his life and mind, and what he later wrote about in psychoanalysis. Reik was afraid that the Baron's fate would become his own, and this became translated into a fear of causing Ella's death. Schnitzler's work fit in precisely with Reik's fear obsessions with death, especially as these were connected to a love relationship. The printed word itself, especially in literature he admired, exerted an almost magical power over Reik's thoughts and feelings.

Stamon and Lawson have recently called attention to the prominence of "Love-Death Structures in the Works of Arthur Schnitzler,"[82] and it is abundantly clear that this element in Schnitzler's work impressed Reik beyond any other. His writing of the two articles on unconscious death wishes and on the omnipotence of thought in Schnitzler took place in the year before his marriage to Ella, and this approaching event must have heavily influenced his focus on these themes.

In a number of places in *Fragment* Reik reiterates that he is providing merely the "fragment" of a confession. "He who reveals himself in some facts makes it easy for himself to conceal certain other personal matters which he may wish to keep secret."[83] The significant fact that Reik withheld was that Maria had already borne his child and that the child was two years old when he went to see Freud.[84] Reik went to Freud not only for help with neurotic symptoms but also for advice and rescue from his actual marital dilemma. In fact, the dilemma may well have been the basic cause of his symptoms. If Reik stayed with Ella, he would be neglecting his duty to Maria and his young child and his feelings for them. But how could he leave Ella, who was now an invalid and dependent upon him? In addition, Ella had by then learned of Maria and the baby, and their marriage had become troubled and stormy. Ella called Reik a scoundrel and other less flattering names, and his conflict was acute and unbearable.

Seen in this light, Freud's comments may be given an interpretation other than that of Reik's idea of his unconscious death wishes. Schnitzler's *Murderer* does indeed provide a number of parallels between Alfred in that story and Theodor Reik. Both were burdened with invalid women who were dependent upon them and whose death would permit a long-desired marriage to another woman. The important difference was that in Schnitzler's story the doctor told Alfred that sex would be dangerous to Elise, whereas Reik had been told by his physician that Ella would *not* be harmed by sex. In a certain sense, Schnitzler's novel was more real to Reik than his actual life situation. Reik maintained that sex was harmful to Ella despite what the doctor told him and despite the fact that Ella "seemed in a subtle way to encourage my lovemaking. . . . There had been no sexual relations between us for a long time."[85]

It is, of course, possible that Reik was correct in his judgment of the bad effects of sex on Ella, in spite of the doctor's opinion and in spite of Ella's own encouragement. However, Freud may have been trying to point out to Reik that Ella, like Elise, would have preferred to die while being loved by her husband rather than being actually neglected or abandoned by him.

In *The Murderer* Elise's wish to continue lovemaking despite her illness is clear and, in fact, a key aspect of the story, and it is significant that this part of a rather transparent plot did not register on Reik. Freud's remarks seem to have been directed toward pointing out to Reik this probable correspondence between Elise's wishes and what Ella may well have wished. Reik's writing in *Fragment* indicates no awareness of what Freud seems to have intended.

The plot of *The Murderer* has implications for both libidinal and aggressive instincts. It was mainly the aggressive death wishes to which Reik responded. Reik's own attachment to Maria and his responsibility to a very young child seem to have turned him toward Maria and away from Ella, and it may have been this situation, not disclosed in *Fragment,* that sensitized Reik to death wishes in Schnitzler's narrative rather than to libidinal ones. It is also possible that in fathering a child outside of marriage Reik was in part expressing an identification with Schnitzler or with the romantic ideal he represented in Reik's mind.[86]

Freud's comment that he "would have thought [Reik] stronger," may also be given further interpretation. Freud might well have intended his remark to mean that Reik should have been strong enough to have prevented such a crisis in his life or even to have resolved the problem on his own without developing the symptoms that led him to ask Freud's help. Freud appears to have been reacting to Reik's excessive dependency upon him.

Freud's question had been aimed at Reik's unconscious guilt feelings with the hope of releasing them to consciousness. Reik did achieve insight into his death wishes toward Ella and also, as a pyschoanalyst, realized that there must have been unconscious guilt.[87] However, he did not actually experience the guilt consciously, as he did the death wish. What seems to have been an intellectual insight, as described in his 1913 article, was changed into an emotional insight by the fact of his actual experiencing of the feeling of wanting Ella to die.[88] Freud tried to get Reik to respond to his wife's own emotional needs, but he was too focused internally to do so.

Freud may also have been disappointed in Reik from an ordinary moral viewpoint, all aside from the notion of the unconscious. Rieff is undoubtedly correct in saying that Freud had the "mind of a moralist,"[89] and Reik was here evading an intrinsically moral problem and in fact doing so in the guise of developing psychoanalytic insight. He was unable to face up to his own responsibility to Ella and shifted this responsibility to Freud, psychoanalysis, and unconscious death wishes.

From a psychoanalytic viewpoint this does not seem to have been a deliberate evasion on Reik's part. Rather, it appears as a form of repression in which Reik's behavior was the direct result of an acute instinctual conflict in which he had no clear awareness of his actions and their consequences. In such troubled times Reik turned to literature, such as that of Schnitzler, and here he found succor in the themes of love, death, and the omnipotence of thoughts—themes that externalized the turmoil he felt within himself. In Freud and psychoanalysis Reik also perceived Eros, Thanatos, and the power of the unconscious. With the help of these powerful allies—Schnitzler and Freud—he was able to live life as if it were a kind of literature. Reik's mode of romanticizing his actual relationship with Ella may be seen in the way he changed even the title of his original Goethe monograph from *Why Did Goethe Leave Friederike?* to *Goethe's Romance with Friederike.* Reik himself acknowledges changing this title but merely says that it had been criticized by a colleague and was "a silly title!"[90]

Freud's question, at the very instant Reik heard it, produced an almost uncanny palliative effect. The question revived once more the theme of thought-murder that had obsessed Reik for many years. It was like an old companion who brought the nostalgic relief of long familiarity. "I heard myself say, 'Oh, that is it?' "[91] After Reik heard the question, he first experienced the actual wish for Ella's death (based in part, possibly, upon an identification with Alfred in Schnitzler's story) and recognized that his previous obsessions had concealed this wish.

If Reik had become aware of Ella's own wishes and needs for him, as Freud seems to have intended, he would have experienced guilt but not the death wish itself. Reik may thus have developed as much insight as was psychologically feasible for him—enough to free him from his symptoms and for the future. And it may well be that Reik here illustrates the realistic limits of insight available to any psychoanalytic patient—the rock bottom choices in life that are uncovered in the intensive psychotherapy relationship.

It is astonishing to realize how many years Reik had lived with the *concept* of unconscious death wishes toward his wife without actually *experiencing* them as such. Despite the explicitness of his obsessions, and despite such writings of his own as *The Unknown Murderer,*[92] Reik did not gain emotional insight until his total life situation permitted the changes that would follow. It was not until Reik was emotionally ready to leave Ella and was able to feel supported by Freud in this decision that insight arrived.

Fortified by this insight and acceptance of his death wish, Reik felt again able to confront Ella. They agreed to part, and Reik's anxiety symptoms gradually left him. In the end Reik did leave Ella, as Goethe had left Friederike, but he did not acknowledge this and tried to disguise its occurrence in his writing. Two years later, in April 1937, Ella died from the illness from which she had long suffered.

Freud's question helped Reik overcome both his symptoms and marital dilemma but perhaps not in the way Freud had intended. Although Freud may have been disappointed in Reik, this did not interfere significantly with their relationship, which continued to be a warm and friendly one.

To summarize, Freud's question and subsequent acceptance of Reik were initially helpful to him for three reasons: (1) Without so intending, Freud helped Reik to continue to avoid facing the problem of his actual moral guilt.[93] (2) Reik was helped because Freud did not condemn him or even insist upon clarifying the issue. He tried gently to lead Reik to this problem, but when Reik continued to be unclear, Freud was content to leave the guilt unconscious. This was an enormous support to Reik because it helped him justify his own behavior to himself, something he was having much difficulty doing. (3) The question and its resolution helped Reik to continue to perceive his own life in literary and mythic dramatic terms.

There is a strange paradox in the fact that Reik first wrote about his "unconscious death wishes" toward Ella in 1913, says in *Fragment* (1949) that he was tormented by these obsessive wishes for many years until his analysis with Freud in 1935, but neglects to mention his original insight of 1913. Apparently Reik repressed this insight both in his analysis with Freud and again in writing *Fragment*. If this omission were simply an intentional evasion, why did Reik mention the originally anonymous article to begin with? Since Reik himself states that he has specifically translated the 1913 article for an abbreviated account in *Fragment* but is "omitting only some unessential points"[94] (*sic*), one can only conclude that he (1) was at least partly aware of the omission, (2) was calling attention to it, and (3) somehow wished to be discovered in this inconsistency.

Further, the "curative" value of the insight Reik achieved with Freud emerges as dubious because the unconscious death wishes surfaced again in Reik's marriage with Maria.

> A few years later [after this second marriage] . . . the first symptoms of a serious illness were observed with Maria. . . . It was not accidental that I had my coronary attack a few days after her death. I know that I must often have wished that she should die.[95]

Reik's insights into his death wishes were only momentary in an emotional sense and soon became repressed again, as he recognized.[96] However, the insight continually re-emerged in an intellectual and obsessive form and was repeatedly described in Reik's writing. This repetitive pattern casts doubt upon Freud's initial concept of insight as a way of truly resolving repression. In Reik's case the repression of death wishes continued to exist throughout his life, as did his constant dwelling upon them. The form of the repression-insight shifted from intellectual rumination to brief emotional experiences and back again, and this may well be true of many people's insights. Thus, insight itself may be a part of the repressive process. One gets the impression that the resolution of Reik's conflict was one of destiny rather than decision. Insight and choice were secondary to the forms and forces that carried Reik onward.

Reik himself may emerge here in an unflattering light, but one gathers that this would not have been uncongenial to him. In his own lifetime Reik tended constantly to provoke controversy, dissent, and even rejection, especially by medical psychoanalysts. Reik's reiterated telling of his not being accepted into the New York Psychoanalytic Society illustrates this dwelling upon his feeling of rejection.[97] However, he also said he would "rather be Reik than President of the American Psychoanalytic Association."[98] This type of rejecting reception was essential to Reik, and he seemed to gather a certain enjoyment from it, a kind of *épater le bourgeois*. In a sense, this very essay could be seen as a kind of rejection, provoked by the very materials Reik himself provided.

Nevertheless, beyond this kind of satisfaction in being rejected Reik was seeking to reveal a deeper truth about himself and mankind, a truth about unconscious morality and immorality that has yet to be explored. In Reik's very last book, *The Many Faces of Sex* (1966), he addressed himself to the problem of "Unconscious Morals" and referred specifically to his own unconscious role in the death of Maria, his neglect of her, and his own coronary attack:

> Morals may be a matter of geography, but geography also includes the great dark continent of the unconscious, in which the old laws of morality are as valid as they were in the barbaric times of our remotest ancestors.[99]

Reik saw his psychoanalytic role as that of a creative artist rather than an exact scientist. He found emotional security in literature long before his career in psychoanalysis, and he well recognized that he was embellishing facts and presenting them in a literary way.

He quotes Paul Desharme: "So-called 'bare' facts are often less truthful than impalpable experiences which have been idealized into symbolic form."[100] Reik also quotes Goethe's "phrase that a fact in our life is important not when it is true, but when it is meaningful."[101] In the very last paragraph of *Fragment* he says, "I have shown myself in this book not as I am but as I think I am."

Reik not only wrote literature but also lived it. Books, plays, and music provided the ideal forms that fashioned Reik's character and the roles he took.

> Looking back at this [early] phase of my life, I am astonished at how great the influence of literature, especially of the great poets—as Goethe—was then on the lives of us young men. They not only prepared us for our experiences; they helped to shape them and to give them a certain development.[102]

This is true of all of us, perhaps to a less degree than Reik but not necessarily to a better effect. Literature and the arts provide ideal forms that are desperately needed by everyone. The truth that Reik provides in *Fragment* is not less than would have been given by a simple statement of fact but rather more.

And psychoanalysis itself may well be considered as much a literary form as a science. The actual terms that Freud used to characterize his discoveries—Eros, Oedipus—indicate that he recognized the mythic and dramatic nature of what he had to tell. Writers like Schnitzler provided the actual literature and drama that helped Reik give form and meaning to his own life. Reik's portrayal of his life yields the magic of words and the morality of truth and fiction.

NOTES

1. Theodor Reik, *Fragment of a Great Confession* (New York: Farrar, Straus, 1949), p. 426. Hereafter cited as *Fragment*.
2. Arthur Schnitzler, *The Murderer,* in *Little Novels,* transl. Eric Sutton (New York: Simon & Schuster, 1929), pp. 221-255.
3. In gathering material for Reik's biography, some of these relationships have become illuminated for me. As a psychoanalyst in training, I was a student of Reik, and later a colleague and friend for some years before he died in 1969. Since Reik knew I was preparing his biography, he was kind enough to permit interviews with him and with members of his family. These are some of the sources I draw upon.
4. Bernd Urban, "Vier unveröffentlichte Briefe Arthur Schnitzler an den Psychoanalytiker Theodor Reik," *Modern Austrian Literature,* Vol. 8, 1975, pp. 236-247.

5. Jeffrey B. Berlin and Elizabeth J. Levy, "On the Letters of Theodor Reik to Arthur Schnitzler." See this Special Issue, pp. 109-130.
6. All Schnitzler diary entries which pertain to Freud and psychoanalysis will appear in a volume written by Bernd Urban and Johannes Cremerius, *Die Literaten und Sigmund Freud. Die Rezeption der Psychoanalyse durch deutschsprachige Dichter und Schriftsteller in der ersten Jahrhunderthälfte,* to be published.
7. All diary entries were translated by the late Adolf G. Woltmann.
8. Theodor Reik, *Richard Beer-Hofman* (Leipzig: Sphinx, 1912).
9. Theodor Reik, "Arthur Schnitzler vor dem 'Anatol': Psychoanalytisches," *Pan,* No. 32, June 27, 1912, pp. 899-905.
10. All citations from Reik's letters to Schnitzler are taken from Jeffrey B. Berlin and Elizabeth J. Levy, loc. cit.
11. Reik's letters to Beer-Hofmann are on file at the Houghton Library, Harvard University. They are in part translated and described in Jeffrey B. Berlin and Elizabeth J. Levy, loc. cit.
12. Theodor Reik, *Fragment,* pp. 9-20. Also see Anonymous (Theodor Reik), "Uber die Wirkungen unbewusster Todeswünsche," *Internationale Zeitschrift für ärtzliche Psychoanalyse,* Vol. 2, 1914, pp. 327-353..
13. For a vivid and insightful picture of the Vienna of this period, see Alfred Schick, "The Vienna of Sigmund Freud," *Psychoanalytic Review,* Vol. 55, 1968, pp. 529-551.
14. For complete psychoanalytic bibliographies, see Alexander Grinstein, *The Index of Psychoanalytic Writings,* Vol. 3 (New York: International Universities Press, 1958), pp. 1620-1632. Also see Henry Walter Brann, "Bibliography," in Robert Lindner, ed., *Explorations in Psychoanalysis* (New York: Julian Press, 1953), pp. 289-298.
15. Theodor Reik, *Ritual: Psychoanalytic Studies (1914-1919),* transl. D. Bryan (New York: Farrar, Straus, 1946).
16. Ernest Jones, *The Life and Work of Sigmund Freud,* Vol. 2 (New York: Basic Books, 1955), p. 197.
17. Theodor Reik, *Listening with the Third Ear* (New York: Farrar, Straus, 1948), p. 29. The name of Reik's daughter Miriam was inspired by Beer-Hofmann's *Lullaby for Miriam.* See Theodor Reik, *The Secret Self* (New York: Farrar, Straus & Young, 1953), p. 304.
18. Theodor Reik, *Flaubert und seine "Versuchung des Heiligen Antonius": Ein Beitrag zur Künsterlerpsychologie* (Minden: J. C. C. Bruns, 1912).
19. Letter to Beer-Hofmann of October 8, 1918, transl. Richard and Annabella B. Nelken.
20. Theodor Reik, "Warum verliess Goethe Friederike? Eine psychoanalytische Monographie," *Imago,* Vol. 15, 1929, pp. 400-537.
21. Henri F. Ellenberger, *The Discovery of the Unconscious* (New York: Basic Books, 1970), p. 471.
22. Ernest Jones, *The Life and Work of Sigmund Freud,* Vol. 1 (New York: Basic Books, 1953), p. 94.
23. Ernest Jones, *The Life and Work of Sigmund Freud,* Vol. 2, p. 84.
24. Ernst L. Freud, ed., *The Letters of Sigmund Freud,* transl. Tania and James Stern (New York: Basic Books, 1960), p. 251. Ernest Jones, *The Life and Work of Sigmund Freud,* Vol. 1, p. 346; Vol. 3 (New York: Basic Books, 1957), p. 427.
25. Ernest Jones, *The Life and Work of Sigmund Freud,* Vol. 3, p. 427.
26. Ernst L. Freud, *The Letters of Sigmund Freud,* letter of May 14, 1922, pp. 339-340.
27. Ernest Jones, *The Life and Work of Sigmund Freud,* Vol. 3, p. 84.
28. Arthur Schnitzler, unpublished diary entries of June 27, 1912; January 10, 1915; December 8, 1923.

29. Otto Rank, *The Double: A Psychoanalytic Study,* 1914 (Chapel Hill: University of North Carolina Press, 1971). Robert Rogers, *A Psychoanalytic Study of the Double in Literature* (Detroit: Wayne State University Press, 1970).
30. See note 26.
31. *Fragment, passim,* esp. pp. 7-38.
32. Theodor Reik, *The Secret Self* (New York: Farrar, Straus & Young, 1952), pp. 133-150.
33. Theodor Reik, *Listening with the Third Ear,* p. viii.
34. There are a number of allusions to Anatole France in various of Reik's works. See especially his chapter "Saint Irony," in *The Secret Self,* pp. 161-183.
35. Herman Nunberg and Ernst Federn, eds., *Minutes of the Vienna Psychoanalytic Society,* Vol. 3 (New York: International Universities Press, 1974), pp. 310-319.
36. Arthur Schnitzler, "The Fate of the Baron von Leisenbohg," *Little Novels,* transl. Eric Sutton (New York: Simon & Schuster, 1929), pp. 3-36.
37. Theodor Reik, "Die 'Allmacht der Gedanken' bei Arthur Schnitzler," *Imago,* Vol. 2, 1913, pp. 319-335.
38. Theodor Reik, *The Need to Be Loved* (New York: Farrar, Straus, 1963), pp. 57-59.
39. Arthur Schnitzler, "Redegonda's Diary," *Little Novels,* pp. 181-192.
40. Theodor Reik, *Arthur Schnitzler als Psycholog* (Minden: J. C. C. Bruns, 1913).
41. Theodor Reik, "Das Geschlechterverhältnis bei Schnitzler," *Die neue Generation,* Vol. 9, March 1913, pp. 128-135.
42. Theodor Reik, Review of Arthur Schnitzler, "Frau Beate und ihr Sohn," *Imago,* Vol. 3, 1914, pp. 537-539.
43. Theodor Reik, "Der Tod und die Liebe (In Memoriam Arthur Schnitzler)," *Almanach* (Wien: Internationaler Psychoanalytischer Verlag, 1934), pp. 78-84.
44. Theodor Reik, *The Secret Self,* pp. 151-160. Reik also refers to *Reigen* in *Fragment,* pp. 341-344; *Jewish Wit* (New York: Gamut Press, 1962), p. 101; *The Many Faces of Sex* (New York: Farrar, Straus & Giroux, 1966), p. 193.
45. *Listening with the Third Ear,* p. 32; *Fragment,* p. 342; *Jewish Wit,* pp. 58, 94, 100-101, 230, 239-240.
46. *Fragment,* pp. 225, 304-306; *Of Love and Lust* (New York: Jason Aronson, 1974), p. 426.
47. *Fragment,* pp. 342-344 (translated by Reik as "The Great Buffoon"); *Jewish Wit,* pp. 100-101.
48. *Fragment,* p. 349; *The Secret Self,* pp. 216, 230, 233-234; *Of Love and Lust,* p. 580; *Jewish Wit,* p. 55.
49. Theodor Reik, *Voices from the Inaudible* (New York: Farrar, Straus, 1964), p. 10.
50. *The Secret Self,* pp. 228-229; *The Haunting Melody* (New York: Grove Press, 1953), pp. 149, 221.
51. Theodor Reik, *Pagan Rites in Judaism* (New York: Farrar, Straus, 1964), p. 51.
52. The great classicists, whose work Reik draws upon even more than that of Schnitzler, are Goethe, Shakespeare, and Dostoevsky.
53. "In 1922 Hofmannsthal wrote about Schnitzler's plays '[They are] designed to captivate, to engross, to entertain, and in an ingenious manner to surprise.' " Quoted from Reinhard Urbach, *Arthur Schnitzler,* transl. Donald Daviau (New York: Ungar, 1973), p. 31.
54. *Fragment,* p. 473.

55. Theodor Reik, "Die zweifache Uberraschung," *Die Psychoanalytische Bewegung,* Vol. 1, 1929, pp. 212-227. Abstract in *Psychoanalytic Review,* Vol. 20, 1933, p. 227.
56. Theodor Reik, *Der Uberraschte Psycholog: Ueber Erraten und Verstehen unbewusster Vorgänge* (Leiden: Sijthoff, 1935). *Surprise and the Psychoanalyst: On the Conjecture and Comprehension of Unconscious Processes* (New York: Dutton, 1937).
57. Arthur Schnitzler, "Brief an Dr. Hans Henning," ed. Heinrich Schnitzler, *Neue Rundschau,* Vol. 68, No. 1, 1957, pp. 95-96. Transl. Jeffrey B. Berlin. Schnitzler's last will specifies that the publication of any of his letters must include the complete text.
58. See note 42.
59. See note 37.
60. Maurits Katan, "Schnitzler's 'Das Schicksal der Freiherrn von Leisenbohg,'" *Journal of the American Psychoanalytic Association,* Vol. 17, 1969, pp. 904-926.
61. Robert O. Weiss, "A Study of Psychiatric Elements in Schnitzler's *Flucht in die Finsternis,*" *Germanic Review,* Vol. 33, 1958, pp. 251-275.
62. Reinhard Urbach, *Arthur Schnitzler,* transl. Donald Daviau (New York: Ungar, 1973), p. 19.
63. Sigmund Freud, "On the Universal Tendency to Debasement in the Sphere of Love" (1912), *Standard Edition,* Vol. 11 (London: Hogarth Press, 1957), p. 187.
64. *Ibid.,* p. 180.
65. Sigmund Freud, "Beyond the Pleasure Principle" (1920), *Standard Edition,* Vol. 18 (London: Hogarth Press, 1955), pp. 3-64.
66. This account of Reik's father's death is recounted more fully in Theodor Reik, "Uber die Wirkungen unbewusster Todeswünsche." See this Special Issue, pp. 38-67.
67. See note 20.
68. Some of these data are taken from a diary kept by Ella Reik, kindly made available to me by her son, Arthur Reik.
69. *Fragment,* pp. 359-361.
70. *Fragment,* p. 418.
71. *Fragment,* p. 423.
72. *Fragment,* pp. 425-426, 433.
73. Theodor Reik, *Curiosities of the Self* (New York: Farrar, Straus & Giroux, 1965), p. 52.
74. *Fragment,* pp. 439-440. Reik later quoted this same remark of Freud in German, "Ich hätte sie für stärker gehalten," in *Sex in Man and Woman: Its Emotional Variations* (New York: Farrar, Straus & Cudahy, 1960), p. 236.
75. *Fragment,* pp. 425-426.
76. *Fragment,* pp. 403-404. Reik frequently returns to this theme of moral courage in his writing. He cites Freud's precedent in this respect: "I believe that what enabled *me* to discover the cause of dream-distortion was my moral courage" ("Josef Popper-Lynkeus and the Theory of Dreams," *Standard Edition,* Vol. 19, p. 263). However, Reik has also said that man is a "moral climber" and that "We all live beyond our moral means" (*Masochism in Modern Man,* New York: Farrar, Straus, 1941, pp. 260, 390).
77. See note 12.
78. *Fragment,* p. 331.
79. *Fragment,* pp. 335-337. Reik was also most impressed by Beer-Hofmann's *Graf von Charolais,* first performed in 1905. See *Fragment,* pp. 470-471; *Listening with the Third Ear,* pp. 93-97; *The Secret Self,* pp. 303-304. The central theme of this drama involves the redemption of the actual dead

body of a father by his son. It would appear that this dramatic happening may well have been incorporated into Reik's obsession, since the play was performed at just about the time his father died.

80. See this Special Issue, pp. 55, 58.
81. See note 37.
82. Peggy Stamon and Richard H. Lawson, "Love-Death Structures in the Works of Arthur Schnitzler," *Modern Austrian Literature,"* Vol. 8, 1975, pp. 266-281.
83. *Fragment,* p. 26.
84. See note 3.
85. *Fragment,* p. 452.
86. Schnitzler's son was born the year before his marriage to the child's mother.
87. *Fragment,* pp. 438, 444-446.
88. Reik does not say this explicitly. The statement of Reik's actual experiencing of death wishes is a psychoanalytic "construction." See Sigmund Freud, "Constructions in Analysis" (1937), *Standard Edition,* Vol. 23 (London: Hogarth Press, 1964), pp. 255-269.
89. Philip Rieff, *Freud: The Mind of a Moralist* (New York: Doubleday Anchor Book, 1961).
90. *Fragment,* p. 218.
91. *Fragment,* p. 426.
92. Theodor Reik, *The Unknown Murderer* (1932), transl. Katherine Jones, in *The Compulsion to Confess* (New York: Farrar, Straus & Cudahy, 1959).
93. "I recognized that Freud did not consider my hidden and forbidden impulse . . . from the point of view of morals" (*Fragment,* p. 440). Cf. note 76. This is a manifestly complex problem that cannot be considered further here.
94. *Fragment,* p. 331.
95. Theodor Reik, *Curiosities of the Self,* p. 52.
96. "The removal [of repressions by psychoanalysis] is only temporary, we might say often momentary" (*Listening with the Third Ear,* pp. 492-493).
97. *Fragment,* pp. 319-321, 326-327, 412-415.
98. *Fragment,* p. 318.
99. *The Many Faces of Sex,* pp. 42-43.
100. *Fragment,* p. 63.
101. *Fragment,* p. 35.
102. *Fragment,* p. 314.

350 Central Park West
New York, N.Y. 10025

Special Book Review

KARL KRAUS IN ENGLISH TRANSLATION

Donald G. Daviau

IN THESE GREAT TIMES: A KARL KRAUS READER. Edited by Harry Zohn. Montreal: Engendra Press, 1976. 263 pp.

HALF TRUTHS AND ONE-AND-A-HALF TRUTHS: SELECTED APHORISMS. Edited and translated by Harry Zohn. Montreal: Engendra Press, 1976. 128 pp.

THE LAST DAYS OF MANKIND BY KARL KRAUS. Abridged and edited by Frederick Ungar. New York: Frederick Ungar Publishing Co., Inc., 1974. 263 pp.

NO COMPROMISE: SELECTED WRITINGS OF KARL KRAUS. Edited by Frederick Ungar. New York: Frederick Ungar Publishing Co., Inc., 1977. 260 pp.

KARL KRAUS AND THE SOUL DOCTORS: A PIONEER CRITIC AND HIS CRITICISM OF PSYCHIATRY AND PSYCHOANALYSIS. Thomas Szasz. Baton Rouge: Louisiana State University Press, 1976. 180 pp.

Until recently, Karl Kraus, the Austrian writer, social critic, and Vienna's satirist in residence, was considered to be an untranslatable author. Suddenly, within the space of three years, five works in English translation have appeared, and from these books collectively English-speaking readers can now begin to form some judgment of Kraus and his writings on the basis of a rendition of his own words. Although it perhaps sounds exaggerated, there is in fact a greater difference in reading Kraus in translation than is the case with most other authors. The reason lies in Kraus's extremely rich and complex style. While obviously an author's style is always important, usually the subject matter dominates, and even in the case of a remarkable stylist like Thomas Mann, the content can be acceptably rendered into another language without severe loss, as we know from the brilliant translations of H. Lowe-Porter. In Kraus, however, language itself is often the very substance of his writings. Not only does he use

0033-2836/78/1300-0095 $00.95

highly connotive language, rich in puns, double meanings, and allusions, but his thought is rooted in words that cut in several, sometimes even in opposing directions at the same time. To find English equivalents for individual words is in many cases already a substantial problem, but to maintain this degree of complexity and range of meanings with all of the allusive force of the original throughout an entire paragraph or essay becomes a virtuoso accomplishment, when it is not impossible. For this reason, there are some of Kraus's writings that will forever elude translation, unless one is satisfied with a crude adaptation or approximation of the original rather than a faithful rendering of Kraus's words. Through paraphrase it is possible to gain an idea of what Kraus is writing about, but one will still not have experienced the inimitable Krausian style.

In the various books under discussion here the translators and editors have adopted different approaches to the difficult task of reproducing Kraus in English. I begin with the works edited by Harry Zohn, because to date I feel he is one of the most capable and conscientious translators of Kraus. Zohn, who holds Kraus and his writings in the highest esteem, knows Kraus as well as any scholar writing today. His credentials include the best book on Kraus in English (*Karl Kraus*, New York: Twayne Publishers, 1971), and a considerable gift for language both in English and in German, a talent which serves him well in capturing the nuances of Kraus's word plays and other linguistic complexities. Other translators represented in the volume *In These Great Times* besides Zohn, who translated excerpts from Kraus's journal *Die Fackel,* are Karl F. Ross, who translated a number of poems, and Max Knight and Joseph Fabry, who have translated a stage version of Kraus's magnum opus *The Last Days of Mankind*.

This reader provides a representative overview of most of Kraus's major literary forms and thematic concerns. The volume contains a short but informative introduction by Zohn that is supplemented by a chronology of Kraus's life, eight pages of pictures, and an excellent charcoal sketch of Kraus. Perhaps since his book on Kraus is available in English, Zohn does not try to give a complete survey of Kraus's life and works in his introduction, but instead limits himself to a discussion of the various selections in the volume, providing useful background to afford some broader perspective and also sufficient commentary to make the selections understandable. His hope is, and the case should be, that anyone sampling this reader will be attracted sufficiently to Kraus to want to pursue his reading to the other volumes.

The major notable omission from *In These Great Times* is any selection of Kraus's aphorisms, one of his favorite and most successful forms. The reason is that these are to be found in Zohn's companion volume *Half Truths and One-and-a-Half Truths.* Since neither book is overly large or long, it is not quite clear why they were not combined in order to provide a more comprehensive view of Kraus in one work. It is true that the resulting book would have been more expensive than either of the present volumes, but it would not have been as expensive as the two published separately. Moreover, the introductions of both volumes could have then been more conveniently combined into a fuller portrait of Kraus all in one place. As it is, the Introduction of *Half Truths* provides a general survey of Kraus's life and works and thus supplements rather than duplicates the introduction of *In These Great Times.*

The purpose of *Half Truths* is in Zohn's own words

> to set before English readers a mosaic of Karl Kraus's views, attitudes, and ideas as he disclosed them in aphoristic form, a manner of expression in which Kraus has few peers among modern authors. (p. 2)

The selections cover most of Kraus's main concerns: the follies of his society, the prevailing double standard of morality, and his hatred of the press, which he saw in league with the forces of corruption, dissolution, and decay. In addition, one can see his ambivalent attitude toward the Jews, his pacifism which is magnificently captured in *The Last Days of Mankind,* his polemics against other authors, and against political figures such as police chief Johannes Schober and the corrupt press boss Imre Békessy. Zohn also points out Kraus's fascinating talent as a public performer, giving recitals of his own works as well as performances of Shakespearean plays and Offenbach operettas with himself reading or singing all of the parts. Kraus's attitude toward Hitler and toward Nazism and politics in general in the later years is also discussed, as are his attacks on psychoanalysis and the "psychoanals," as he called psychoanalysts. His hostility to pyschoanalysis stemmed from the belief that it contributed to the crushing of the human spirit and from his fear of its potential for misuse. Above all, Kraus's lifelong crusade for the integrity of language is stressed, the overriding concern that subsumes all of his other ideas.

The aphorism was a natural form for Kraus, for he was not a systematic thinker and never made any attempt to round off his ideas into a total program. It is impossible to categorize Kraus or to pin convenient labels to his writings, for he did not see any virtue in consistency for its own sake. If his thinking led him to what he regarded as a better solution to a problem or if he simply saw things in a different light for whatever reason, the resulting inconsistencies and contradictions in his writings were of little import to him.

One most useful and informative aspect of Zohn's introduction is his effort to point out some of the difficulties in attempting to translate Kraus. By means of a working example that Zohn translates in a variety of ways, he demonstrates effectively the richness of Kraus's imaginative use of language and some of the problems confronting the potential translator. In a very large and true sense the selection of works to be contained in the two volumes has been determined not so much by the editor's wishes as by what he felt could be well translated. As Zohn himself notes:

> Many of the most brilliant and characteristic of Kraus's thousands of aphorisms, especially those dealing with language, imagination, the artistic process, and verbal creativity, have had to be excluded because of their essential untranslatability. (p. 25)

If the two volumes edited by Zohn had been combined, the resulting book would have resembled in scope and in format the anthology *No Compromise* edited by Frederick Ungar. Like Zohn, Ungar is a devoted admirer of Kraus and one of the people in this country who has long desired to see the writings of the great Austrian satirist and critic made available in English. He pioneered efforts in this direction three years ago by publishing an abridged version in English translation of *The Last Days of Mankind.*

Since Ungar's previous volume devoted exclusively to this drama is still in print, it can perhaps be questioned why it was deemed desirable to utilize almost a third of the present volume (89 of 260 pages) in needless duplication. On the one hand it seems a disservice to Kraus to condense his magnificent satire in this manner to a mere skeleton of the original, since its effectiveness depends in large part on a collage effect built up over its many scenes; and on the other hand it seems that this space could have been more advantageously employed for translations of additional material, thus making more of Kraus's work available in English. Moreover, readers of the scenes from *The Last Days of Mankind* contained in *No Compromise* may not feel inclined to acquire the longer but still abridged version of the play. If readers are thus deterred from reading the longer version, they lose in several ways, for they are getting only about ten percent of a play which runs to approximately 770 pages in its original German form, and they are also missing both the informative introduction by Ungar as well as the valuable analysis of the play by Franz Mautner. This perceptive essay helps to overcome the limitations of the abridgment by supplying readers with an evaluation of the total work and by providing information about the scenes that were omitted. Thus readers are able to gain an understanding of the play's extraordinary dimensions, ramifications, and stylistic features, which are not readily apparent in either of the English versions to date. It should be emphasized that while all Kraus's writings are worth knowing, *The Last Days of Mankind* holds special significance, for it is at once Kraus's masterpiece, one of the great dramas of the twentieth century, and perhaps the greatest satiric drama in literature. Moreover, it is one of the most eloquent and effective pacifistic documents ever written.

To prepare the translations for the volume *No Compromise,* Ungar used the services of nine translators including himself. Each of the selections is signed by the translator responsible. In addition, Ungar has written a short introductory essay (fourteen pages) which provides an overview of Kraus's life and activities. Among other topics, he discusses the great sensation that Kraus's initial publication of *Die Fackel* caused in Vienna, the conspiracy of silence (*Totschweigen*) practiced against Kraus by the Viennese press and by other writers, and Kraus's approach to life, which is "aesthetic and ethical and his yardstick the absolute" (p. 8). Kraus's feelings of anti-Semitism and his reactions to World War I are described, as is Kraus's concept of the *Ursprung,* the imaginary ideal source toward which man should be aspiring. Ungar suggests that Kraus's poetry reflects his turn to the timeless realm of nature and from there to the mystery of language as an escape from the horrors of war. Finally,

Ungar briefly discusses *The Last Days of Mankind,* which in his view "is in a way the first documentary drama" (pp. 11-12).

Ungar's introduction overlaps Zohn's to a large degree, and also the selections in *No Compromise* duplicate to some extent those in Zohn's two volumes. While this is unfortunate, it is perfectly understandable, for the choices in both cases were restricted by the material that can be translated. For anyone interested in the general problems of translation in addition to learning about Kraus, it is instructive and engrossing to read the versions of the same text in both volumes, to see how two different translators solve the same problems. Sometimes a given translation seems more successful in Zohn and at other times in Ungar, and on balance it would be difficult to choose between the translations in any of these volumes. The only clear preference would be for the translation of *The Last Days of Mankind* by Alexander Gode and Sue Ellen Wright published by Ungar over the version by Max Knight and Joseph Fabry in the Zohn volume. In general all of the above-mentioned books provide a reasonably good introduction to Kraus's thematic world, and the translations, despite the variations that exist between them, can be recommended on the basis of their conscientious attempt to be as faithful as possible to the intent and language of the original.

Unfortunately, it is not possible to extend this same recommendation to the final volume under review here, *Karl Kraus and the Soul Doctors* by Thomas Szasz. While Zohn is a professor of German with excellent credentials as a scholar and translator and Ungar is a well-known publisher and former Viennese who deserves credit for first breaking the translation barrier with his publication of *The Last Days of Mankind*, Szasz, a professor of psychiatry with at least seven books on psychiatry and mental health to his credit, is here evidently making his first foray into the field of cultural history and translation, to the limited degree that he has actually done either. Unlike the previous books discussed, which have no editorial bias other than an admiration of Kraus and the desire to make his works available and intelligible to English readers, Szasz seems to have written this book primarily as part of a continuing polemic against psychiatry and psychoanalysis. Although Szasz is ostensibly interested in making Kraus known in English, as evidenced by the inclusion of the aphorisms, it soon becomes apparent that his major motivation is not to spread but to trade on Kraus's reputation by enlisting him as an ally to reinforce Szasz's attack on psychiatry and psychoanalysis. In short, this book is not a product of objective scholarship but a subjective diatribe in which Szasz exploits Kraus for his own personal purposes.

It is truly regrettable that Szasz felt impelled to write his book in such aggressive and assertive fashion, because the subjects of psychiatry and psychoanalysis were important concerns of Kraus and to date nothing of consequence has been written about them. A thorough investigation of this aspect of Kraus's thinking and writing, particularly by a man with Szasz's qualifications, could have been a significant and most welcome contribution to the literature about Kraus. However, Szasz is not content merely to have identified a gap in existing scholarship and to proceed to fill it by writing a scholarly book documenting the reasons for Kraus's vehemently articulated rejection of psychiatry and psychoanalysis. Instead, he is convinced that this aspect of Kraus has been purposely avoided, indeed suppressed, and that there has been and still is a world-wide conspiracy of silence against the works of Kraus, particularly with regard to his attacks on "the soul doctors." If one could agree with Szasz's conspiracy idea, then perhaps one could at least understand his aggressive tone and belligerent manner. But even with good will one cannot overlook or forgive his irresponsible methods of making careless, undocumented charges against other scholars and of twisting facts to fit his preconceived ideas.

For example, let us examine the allegation of a conspiracy of silence against Kraus, since it is a thesis dear to Szasz's heart and central to his book. It is a widely known fact that Kraus was indeed the victim of a silent treatment by the press and other writers of his own day. Both Zohn and Ungar stress this fact in their introductions. This tactic, known as *Totschweigen*—literally to kill an individual by refusing to acknowledge his existence—was a means of self-defense by individuals who either did not dare or did not desire to engage Kraus in polemic. This wall of silence was particularly practiced by the *Neue Freie Presse,* Vienna's most influential newspaper and one of Kraus's favorite targets. So thoroughly did this newspaper avoid any reference to Kraus that if one had to rely solely on this source for information about this period, it would never be learned that there was a writer at this time named Karl Kraus.

However, even then *Totschweigen* was not a widespread conspiracy, and it did not prevent countless articles about Kraus from being published, as one can easily document from looking at Otto Kerry's detailed bibliographies of secondary literature on Kraus. But Szasz fails to take these sources into account. In fact, he does not even mention Kerry's bibliographies. Rather, he believes that this conspiracy is being continued not only by the members of his profession but also by literary scholars as well, that it has extended from Europe to America, and that this is the prime reason why Kraus's works have not been translated into English before now. Of course, at the time he was writing his book Szasz was probably unaware that four other volumes of translations were about to be published. However, even this knowledge would most likely have done little to alter Szasz's conviction, because while they do mention Kraus's hostility toward psychiatry and psychoanalysis, neither Zohn nor Ungar discuss the subject in any detail.

Despite all of the comments by qualified scholars like Erich Heller and Heinz Politzer about the difficulties of translating Kraus, Szasz, who has to be considered an amateur as a translator, refuses to accept this viewpoint as the reason why Kraus has not been made available in English before now. Instead, he insists on seeing a conspiracy in action:

> I believe, and I shall try to support my belief with evidence, that he [Kraus] is so little known today because he was on the "wrong" side in the great ideological battle of his time; I further believe that he remains untranslated not so much because his German is so difficult—though it surely is—as because his writings run against the grain of our contemporary mores even more than they did against his. (p. xii)

No one would or could dispute that Kraus's thinking ran counter to that of his age or ours. That is one of the major reasons for his importance and why many scholars have held and continue to hold him up as a model. However, to twist this idea into the cause for the lack of translations of Kraus into English is a misrepresentation that Szasz is unable to prove.

Szasz explains his twofold aim in this book very precisely, namely, to introduce Kraus to the English-speaking public and

> to add a chapter to the history of psychiatry and psychoanalysis—not as such history is usually presented, through the hagiographies

> of "great" psychiatrists, but as it emerges from the work of a contemporary critic of such a great man—in this case Freud—and of his unworthy followers. . . . In short, my aim has been to balance accounts with the psychoanalysts, psychohistorians, and the other tellers of the glorious tale of psychoanalysis who have brutally torn the figure of Karl Kraus from the group portrait of intellectual Vienna during the first third of the century; who, in other words, have tried to erase from the history books Kraus's contributions to modern ideas generally and to the understanding of psychiatry and psychoanalysis specifically. (pp. xii-xiii)

I cannot speak for the psychiatrists and psychologists, who may be ignoring Kraus in their literature, as Szasz alleges, but I can state with some assurance that the idea of all German scholars capable of translating Kraus joining in a conspiracy to prevent such translations is so silly as not to warrant further comment. Since critics of Kraus cannot even agree on whether he was a saint or a devil, it is doubtful that they would agree on anything else about him. If there is any agreement at all, it is in the wish of both groups to air their side of the controversy.

Szasz correctly maintains that Kraus warned against the dangers of psychiatry and psychoanalysis and that these concerns were among his lifelong interests, but it is not true that he presented a "systematic criticism" of these disciplines. As both Zohn and Ungar have stressed in their introductions, Kraus was not a systematic thinker at all, and he altered his views without a qualm, if necessary because of a changed perception of the world and his position in it. He would not have been capable of serving truth as he saw it, if he had not also been capable of changing his mind. If Szasz means continuing criticism, then I could agree with him, but "systematic" is not an apt description for any of Kraus's criticism.

To prove his theory of a conspiracy Szasz adduces only weak evidence, such as the fact that there was only one notice in the American press of the symposium held in Vienna in 1974 to commemorate the Kraus centennial. However, if one stops to realize that in 1974 there was nothing of Kraus available in English translation, and that his name, in the absence of any available texts, was not known to the public, there seems to have been little reason for American newspapers to take cognizance of this event. Surprisingly (or really not so in view of the few German sources Szasz seems to know), in his discussion of this conference Szasz does not make any mention of the book by Helmut Arntzen, who has analyzed this conference in a much more scholarly and persuasive fashion in his work *Karl Kraus und die Presse* (Munich: Fink Verlag, 1975). Since Arntzen believes that the *Totschweigen* tactic is still being perpetuated today by the media because of Kraus's exposures of its evils, Szasz would have found a useful ally. However, he would probably not be interested in any conspiracy but his own. One must always be careful in understanding Szasz's particular meaning of words. For Szasz *Totschweigen* is selective:

> The rule is the *Totschweigentaktik*—directed, to be sure, not toward Kraus's person or work in general, as it had been in the days of the *Neue Freie Presse,* but, selectively, towards his criticisms of psychiatry and psychoanalysis, as befits the days of the *New York Review.* The special Karl Kraus issue of *Modern Austrian Literature,* published in 1975, is illustrative. Although Donald Daviau, the Editor, promises a collection of essays that "touches upon major aspects of Kraus's thought, attitudes, and activities," he delivers one in which there is only a single brief, and quite misleading, reference to Kraus's lifelong preoccupation with, and opposition to, the soul doctors." (p. 88)

This sample of Szasz's single-mindedness and willful misreading provides a good insight into his methods. As can be seen here, it is not sufficient that one attempt to publicize Kraus; unless one specifically stresses Kraus's views on psychoanalysis, he is guilty of participating in the conspiracy to perpetuate the silent treatment. Szasz not only accuses me of failing to deliver what I promised, but by juxtaposing this charge to the previous sentence, as seen above, he also uses innuendo to create the suspicion that I must have willfully refrained from publishing any manuscripts that would have touched upon the subjects of interest to Szasz. This turns out in fact to be a flagrant example of selective quotation that shows clearly how Szasz maliciously twists my words to suit his purpose. The sentence that I actually wrote gives a totally different impression: "The collection of essays presented here is eclectic, but it nevertheless touches upon major aspects of Kraus's thought, attitudes, and activities."*

* Special Karl Kraus issue, *Modern Austrian Literature,* Vol. 8, Nos. 1/2, 1975, p. 8.

Szasz could not mistake the meaning of this full sentence, and therefore his irresponsible tactics here illustrate to what lengths he will go to prove himself right and everyone else wrong.

Szasz's book is divided into two parts: Part I (one hundred pages) contains five chapters, the titles of which provide a good overview of the contents: "The Man and His Work," "Kraus and Freud: Unmasking the Unmasker," "Karl Kraus: Noble Rhetorician," "Kraus's Place in Cultural History," and "Kraus Today." The second part of the book (sixty pages) contains selected translations from Kraus's aphoristic writings under the following headings: "On Psychoanalysis and Psychology," "On Institutional and Forensic Psychiatry," and "On Language, Life, and Love." The book contains no bibliography of secondary sources, and the references in the Notes barely go beyond the few major sources in English, particularly Harry Zohn and Wilma Iggers, interestingly enough, two of the better Kraus scholars whom Szasz spends much of his time attacking, while at the same time relying heavily on their scholarship in the writing of his book. Szasz's first chapter, for example, with its survey of Kraus's life and works, contains nothing that could not have been borrowed from Zohn or Iggers. A bibliography of Kraus's works is dropped into the text (p. 15), but it loses some of its usefulness because the various titles are not identified by genre. At the end of the list Szasz merely notes in general that "These volumes contain prose and poetry, plays and aphorisms."

In the chapter on Kraus and Freud, Szasz refutes the claim that Kraus turned against psychoanalysis after the attack on him by Fritz Wittel on January 12, 1910, in a paper delivered before the Vienna Society. Szasz analyzes Wittel's paper and also Freud's affirmative reaction to it, which shows how the two great rhetoricians Freud and Kraus were diametrically opposed in their intellectual outlook:

> As Freud wrote some of the greatest apologetics of our age for a science of man and his mental life, so Kraus wrote some of the greatest apologetics of it for the dignity and individuality of the person as a moral agent. This made them adversaries in the grandest tradition of rhetoric: men struggling for what each sees as salvation, and for what his adversary sees as damnation. (p. 41)

Using terminology borrowed from Richard Weaver, Szasz then defines Kraus as a noble rhetorician and Freud as a base rhetorician.

According to Weaver, base rhetoric is "speech which influences us in the direction of evil" (p. 53), while

> The noble rhetorician uses language to wean men away from their inclination to depend on authority, to encourage them to think and speak clearly, and to teach them to be their own masters,

as Szasz paraphrases Weaver (p. 54). Once Szasz has established his criteria, it is an easy matter to use Kraus as a club with which to beat Freud and psychoanalysis.

It is not possible in the space of a review to note all of the instances where Szasz distorts and finesses evidence to support his ideas. A few more examples will have to suffice. A case in point is the issue Szasz takes with the judgment of most scholars that despite his achievements Kraus was a failure. He cites Zohn's conclusion to his biography of Kraus as a typical judgment. Zohn writes:

> In his inability to save his time by turning his fellow men to the sources of spiritual power in their cultural heritage, in his fighting a rear guard action in behalf of a spirit of a dying age, in his relentless, truculent criticism of so many aspects of human nature, Kraus may have been a failure. But surely he was one of the grandest failures in world literature. (p. 56)

Now any objective person reading this rhetorical culmination to Zohn's laudatory biography cannot fail to recognize that Zohn does not think that Kraus was a failure at all. Yet Szasz, ever intent on criticizing his predecessors at any cost, the better to prove himself as the White Knight come to save Kraus from the infidels, totally ignores Zohn's meaning and the context in which the statement is made. Instead, he establishes a totally different criterion than Zohn had been using, in order to contradict Zohn and show that Kraus was successful after all. Using such a "bait and switch tactic," as Szasz does here, is a sample of the unfair argumentative technique Szasz employs to "prove" his case.

Another unscholarly method that Szasz uses is to finesse his argument rather than to provide solid evidence. The best example occurs in Szasz's attempt to prove Kraus's influence on Egon Friedell, author of the esteemed *Cultural History of the Modern Age*. Szasz states: "Of more importance to us here than his favorable opinion of Kraus and his work is Friedell's opinion of Freud and psychoanalysis. His views on this subject were *probably* influenced by Kraus" (p. 70, emphasis added). No evidence is presented to substantiate this claim of influence, but the entire section on Friedell and Kraus is written as if the probability were fact. To assert connections of this kind without proof is not scholarship. Kraus may well have influenced Friedell, but the task of proving it remains to be done.

These examples should suffice to show how Szasz manipulates facts and hence to warn readers against accepting any of Szasz's evidence or findings at face value. As it stands, his book is unreliable and can serve only two useful functions: it will call attention to Kraus, which is desirable, and it should serve as a provocation to others to rewrite this chapter of Kraus's life and activities in an objective, fair-minded, and scholarly manner.

It is as surprising as it is paradoxical that Szasz, who has written his book ostensibly to make a case for the dignity of man, seems to demonstrate so little understanding of what that means. In his final summary Szasz includes the following words:

> Kraus felt that a civilized person's first obligation was just that—being civil. To him this meant that such a person had an irrefragable obligation to practice the ethic of respect, not only toward persons but towards crafts and traditions as well. (p. 162)

This plea for an "ethic of respect" toward others after the practices he has engaged in throughout his book gives these sentences an ironic twist that would be humorous, if it were not so pathetic. By the glaring descrepancy between his idealistic aims and his unethical methods of argument Szasz has made himself the kind of target that Kraus sought out and attacked all his life.

Concerning his translations of Kraus's aphorisms, Szasz readily acknowledges that he himself is not "the translator" but that he had the assistance of his brother George, of Marcel Faust, a Viennese-American scholar, and of his mother. Szasz assembled the translations prepared by his family and friend and then rendered the sense and the content into English. Szasz is at least candid enough to admit that his mastery of the German language, "good enough in my youth, has declined over decades of non-use" (p. 17). His aim was

> not a slavish, and surely not a verbatim, translation of the Krausian text. That would be a hopeless task for a translator faced with any author, certainly with any German author, and obviously with Kraus, who was a superb aphorist and a great player on and with words. (p. xviii)

Thus, although a few pages earlier Szasz had minimized the difficulties of translating Kraus (p. xii), he now states categorically that a translation would in fact be a hopeless task. What he does present then is not a translation at all but an adaptation or, as he puts it, his "aim was to transmute Kraus's thought and spirit into clear and idiomatic—and, where appropriate, pungent and ironic—English" (p. xviii). One need only compare Szasz's adaptation of these aphorisms to the translations in the other volumes in order to see the difference between the two forms. All the aphorisms rendered into Szasz's English versions still require accurate translation.

Since I have devoted more space to reviewing Szasz's book than to the other four volumes, the reasons should perhaps be noted briefly. For one thing, the nature of the volumes edited by Zohn and Ungar—anthologies and translation—is different from the type of argumentative book written by Szasz, and for another the quality varies sharply. When it is necessary to criticize a book, I feel that it is the obligation of the reviewer not merely to assert what is wrong but also to document such claims with solid textual proof. This procedure requires greater length, which accounts for the disproportionate space distribution here.

In summary, a good beginning can be seen here to the task of making the writings of Karl Kraus available in English. It seems certain that others will be attracted to follow this lead and that additional translations as well as critical and interpretative works on Kraus will be forthcoming. The situation looks most encouraging for the day when Kraus will receive the recognition in English-speaking countries that he merits for the ethical and aesthetic contributions he has made to Western thought, literature, and culture.

University of California
Riverside, Ca. 92521

ON THE LETTERS OF THEODOR REIK TO ARTHUR SCHNITZLER

Jeffrey B. Berlin and Elizabeth J. Levy

For Heinrich Schnitzler*

In his article "Reik and the Interpretation of Literature," A. Bronson Feldman suggests that "the analysis of Schnitzler's masterpieces and ephemeral writings was typical of Reik's way of handling the geniuses he idolized."[1] Reik expressed such a view in *Fragment of a Great Confession,* where he writes: "My admiration for the great gift of psychological observation of a contemporary Viennese writer was expressed in *Arthur Schnitzler as Psychologist* (1913)."[2] Reik's interest in Schnitzler (1862-1931) was not confined to this book. He also wrote several articles on Schnitzler's works and even reviewed *Frau Beate and Her Son.*[3] Reik originally intended to dedicate his *Arthur Schnitzler as Psychologist* to Schnitzler (see letter 2), but it is unknown if Schnitzler denied him permission. The work carries the statement: "Dedicated to my admired teacher Professor Dr. Sigmund Freud in gratitude."[4]

Occasionally Reik's comments illuminate aspects of Schnitzler's personality; for example, Reik observes in *The Need To Be Loved*: "A psychoanalytic investigation into Schnitzler's plays and novels would

* We wish to acknowledge our gratitude to Arthur Reik for his kind permission to publish his father's letters and for making available the Beer-Hofmann letters to his father. The original Reik letters to Schnitzler are deposited at the University Library in Cambridge, England, along with much of the posthumous papers of Arthur Schnitzler. We thank Reinhard Urbach for calling our attention to them. We also thank Miriam Beer-Hofmann Lens for her permission to publish her father's letters, as well as for making available Reik's letters to herself. The Reik letters to Beer-Hofmann are deposited at the Harvard College Library and are reproduced by the permission of the library.

0033-2836/78/1300-0109 $00.95 © 1978 N.P.A.P.

lead to the impression that the writer, as a mature man, had paranoic ideas of various kinds."[5] Reik continues:

> Just now I recall some memories of Schnitzler, whom I had known for many years. We often took walks on the Sommerheidenweg near Vienna and I vividly remember that our conversation moved from general topics to personal things, and that he sometimes revealed suspicious thoughts and paranoic tendencies.[6]

And in *Fragment of a Great Confession* Reik claims: "There were not many people in Vienna who knew the writings of Schnitzler as well as I."[7]

For several reasons, then, it is not surprising that references to Schnitzler's works are often found in Reik's books, which serve to clarify Reik's position or to demonstrate a parallel situation.[8] In *Fragment of a Great Confession,* for example, Reik draws a sagacious parallel between Goethe's story of Lucinde's curse and Schnitzler's Kläre in *The Fate of the Baron von Leisenbohg.*[9] In another instance we learn that Freud, who considered Schnitzler his "double,"[10] had referred to a Schnitzlerian work (*The Murderer*) during an analytic session with Reik to suggest the nature of Reik's unconscious guilt. In this regard, Murray H. Sherman, in a discerning article, observes that "actually, Freud's allusion, as Reik spells out the plot of *The Murderer,* has implications for both the libidinal and aggressive instincts, but Reik seems to have responded mainly to the death wish implications."[11] It is interesting to observe, incidentally, that Reik affirms that Freud considered Schnitzler his "double," and it is regretful that Reik offered no further elucidation of this statement in his interviews with Erika Freeman.[12] Nevertheless, Anna Freud clarified this latter point very succinctly in a letter to this writer:

> There is no difficulty in explaining what my father meant when he used the word *Doppelgänger.* He often spoke about the fact that poets and writers in their own way come to the same conclusions about human nature as he had to fight for in painstaking analytical work with patients. In this sense, therefore, the novelist is the double (*Doppelgänger*) of the analyst.[13]

Until the recent publication of four Schnitzler letters to Reik, which were edited with extensive notes by Bernd Urban,[14] little attention had been given to their personal relationship. Reik knew

Schnitzler personally. In *Voices from the Inaudible: The Patients Speak*, for example, Reik writes: "My son is named after Schnitzler, who took some interest in the boy. We lived in Vienna in the Sternwartestrasse—as did Arthur and Olga Schnitzler, who sometimes invited me to dinner at their hospitable home."[15] And in *Listening with the Third Ear* Reik, searching his own thoughts, writes:

> The photograph of Arthur Schnitzler . . . I remember him and I see him as I took a walk with him in Vienna on the Sommerhaidenweg. . . . We lived in the same street and my son was named after him. . . . I once wished that Arthur would become a writer like Arthur Schnitzler, whom I loved. . . . Schnitzler was a physician but he left his practice because he preferred writing. . . . I hoped my son would study medicine.[16]

Although more information is now available, Feldmann's perceptive remarks proposed in 1953 still adequately summarize what may be the major significance of Schnitzler for Reich:

> The hankering for a physician's career remained at the back of Reik's mind, and so he came to respect in Arthur Schnitzler the model of the man he might have been: the doctor of medicine, the nonpareil psychologist, the artist in prose.[17]

Schnitzler critics view the situation differently. Robert O. Weiss maintains that

> Dr. Reik's book shows one thing: Arthur Schnitzler's figures are so real, so penetratingly conceived, and so truly represented that as a professional psychoanalyst Reik could not resist practicing his skill on them.[18]

Indeed, Reik's *Arthur Schnitzler as Psychologist* has remained a standard reference work for Schnitzler scholars. Despite the fact that not all critics agree with Reik's approach to literature, they cannot deny the accuracy of his observations.[19] As a matter of fact, Schnitzler himself commented on Reik's book in a letter to Hans Henning dated April 2, 1914:

> It is understandable that I do not like to discuss writings that concern me. This time it is all the more difficult, because I know Dr. Reik personally, hold him in high esteem, and, furthermore, have made no secret of the fact, either before or after the publication of

> his book, that I have scruples about the onesidedness of the psychoanalytical method practiced by him and other students of Freud, regardless of the very interesting and sometimes even correct results it may lead to. Then, too, because I have been asked to express an opinion to you, a man who has the intention of writing about the Reik book himself and in this connection, like it or not, about me as well. I would therefore prefer to limit my remarks from an author's point of view to those aspects of Theodor Reik's presentation which seem to me likeable and valuable in a larger context: Reik draws attention to something that certain professional critics usually ignore: namely, my depiction of non-erotic human relationships as between siblings, parents and children, and friends. He also points out various deeper psychological connections, though he does not exactly say the last word about them and in some cases probably is not absolutely correct. In addition, from conversations with Reik (no more than two or three thus far) I have gained the conviction (though he still has not) that in the future he will look upon Freud's methods of interpretation (regardless of the depth of knowledge of human nature from which the basic ideas might originally have emerged) not as the sole and only path to salvation, but as one among many that leads to the secret of poetic creation, at times, however, into vagueness or error. Surely you will be kind enough to send me your critique when it is available. For now let me thank you most cordially for your kind interest.[20]

Reik's interest in Schnitzler, which began at age eighteen,[21] never receded. He was among the first members of the International Arthur Schnitzler Research Association when it was founded in 1961 and remained a member until his death in 1969.[22] In New York, where he settled, Reik often met with Richard Beer-Hofmann (1866-1945).[23] Beer-Hofmann, a member of the "Jung-Wien" group[24] like Schnitzler, was also revered by Reik, possibly even more than Schnitzler was.[25] In addition to their trusting and cordial relationship, each probably served the other as a remembrance of their days in Vienna.[26] Beer-Hofmann was one of Schnitzler's closest friends and was even named by Schnitzler as one of the executors of his literary estate.[27] It seems quite plausible that Schnitzler would sometimes become the subject of their conversations when Reik visited Beer-Hofmann at his home in New York.[28]

Owing to the bond that existed between Reik, Beer-Hofmann, and Schnitzler, it is valuable to consider, even if only briefly, the basic attitude Reik held toward Beer-Hofmann. Their relationship, in fact, becomes all the more meaningful in consideration of newly discovered

letters, particularly when these are examined in respect to Reik's many comments about Beer-Hofmann in his books. To be sure, this aspect of Reik's personality has also received too little critical attention.

To begin, consider Reik's first encounter with Beer-Hofmann's works, as expressed by Reik in *Fragment of a Great Confession*:

> I first heard the name [of Beer-Hofmann] when I was eighteen, and shortly after my father's death I had read his *Graf von Charolais* [see letter 10]. I was deeply moved. Here was a poet, a real poet, of incomparable power of expression and riches of the heart. My first book, a small pamphlet, was on the work of Beer-Hofmann.[29] I was twenty-three when I wrote it and full of pride when I showed the first copy to Ella. On the first page stood the words *cum ira et studio,* because I was then full of indignation about the Vienna critics who did not give full appreciation to Beer-Hofmann, and very keen to show how wonderful the *Graf von Charolais* and *Schlaflied für Miriam*[30] were. That was 1911.[31]

Clearly the young Reik was proud of his forty-four page booklet. In a letter dated March 4, 1912, Reik wrote to Beer-Hofmann:

> As I send you the enclosed small essay, I should very much like, my dear Herr Doctor, to thank you for the pleasure which your works have often given me. I don't know to what extent I have succeeded in expressing that which many have found in them—my attempt was an honest one. And it seemed to me as if some of it had to be expressed in the face of ignorant critics and an ignorant public.[32]

The next year, in a letter dated June 24, 1913, Reik comments to Beer-Hofmann:

> As promised, I am sending you today the section from my study about Schnitzler. I do not believe that a forcible connection is made in it, but rather that a compelling connection is being demonstrated. If there is any merit in that, the major part is owed to psychoanalysis.[33]

Twenty-one years later, when Reik was in The Hague, he wrote to Beer-Hofmann:[34]

> Your friendly note has made me feel really ashamed; I thank you most kindly for the poems you sent. I purchased *Der junge David* immediately after its publication and luxuriated for many days in

its beauty. I am pleased that in my lecture yesterday I was able to interest many young people in your works which, as one's initial reading of them recedes in time, keep increasing in stature as if the experience embodied in them gradually and slowly rose to the surface. I wish you could have seen the looks of profound emotion in their eyes and faces when later on I read to them the two poems and several scenes from the *Count of Charolais*. Perhaps the love of your poetry made up for what I lacked in the art of delivery. At any rate, I succeeded in getting many people to turn to your books.[35]

Without doubt, then, Beer-Hofmann also played an important role in Reik's life. He served as a friend, admirer, and counselor in both Europe and the United States (see letter 13 and note 61). But, even more, Beer-Hofmann's works, like Schnitzler's, were a source of emotional release for Reik's own poetic and analytical inspirations. Similarly, Beer-Hofmann's works gave Reik hope and sustained him in time of troubles. (Reik was drafted into the Austrian army in January 1915 and served until November 1918. A brief account of some of his army experiences is offered in *The Search Within*.[36]) To be sure, Reik's comments to Beer-Hofmann in a letter of May 18, 1916, are very similar to those written to Schnitzler on the same day (see letter 10):

Many thanks for your kind postcard that I received belatedly because I was transferred and had a new mailing address. I am on horseback almost all day. It would make me very happy if you permitted me to visit you again when I return—if I return. *The Count of Charolais*, which I have with me, has given me something like comfort and tranquillity in these days, as oftentimes before.[37]

The next month, on June 4, 1918, Reik wrote to Beer-Hofmann:

I am just reading in the newspaper that we shall have the *Count of Charolais* in Vienna—probably forever. I am very happy about that. Here one sometimes experiences such dreadful things that one believes it will never be possible to laugh again.[38]

Along with Freud and Mahler, then, Beer-Hofmann and Schnitzler clearly were significant figures to Reik, as he further indicates in *Fragment of a Great Confession*:

They are all dead now, all the men who had meant so much to my

> youth in Vienna. The pictures of Freud, Schnitzler, Mahler, and Beer-Hofmann on the walls of my room do not greet me any more. . . . Why do I suddenly feel so lonely?[39]

As noted, Bernd Urban's publication of some of Schnitzler's letters to Reik establishes a relationship that was previously unknown. He indicates, for example, that Schnitzler met Reik at a time when the former was most concerned with psychoanalysis.[40] Urban relates that

> Schnitzler's letters . . . are of . . . importance in so far as they reveal the approval and criticism of a concerned person of a practice which at that time emanated from the psychoanalysts like a tidal wave: namely, the psychoanalytic interpretation of literature and biography.[41]

The present publication is not intended as a critical assessment of the relationship between Reik and Schnitzler. It is offered to further clarify their association with each other. These nineteen newly discovered letters from Reik to Schnitzler, published here for the first time, date from 1912 to 1929. They testify primarily to the importance of Schnitzler for Reik and, secondly, they help clarify several aspects of Reik's earliest days in Vienna. The Reik letters to and from Beer-Hofmann are also published here for the first time.

[*1*]

VIENNA, 2 July 1912

DEAR HERR DOCTOR,[42]

Your so very gracious note has embellished a summer evening that threatened to become quite melancholy, with a deeply and sincerely felt joy.

I shall be in Vienna once more during the first weeks of September, and will then take the liberty to accept your gracious invitation, for which I thank you most heartily.

With sincere respect
Very devotedly yours
THEODOR REIK

[2]

VIENNA, 25 July 1913

DEAR HERR DOCTOR,

My book about you has now been completed[43] and this autumn is to be issued by J. C. Bruns, which published my Flaubert.[44]

I am taking the liberty to ask, dear Herr Doctor, if I may dedicate it to you.[45] Your permission would give me great joy.[46]

With deep respect
Very devotedly yours
THEODOR REIK

[3]

VIENNA, 20 December 1913

MY DEAR HERR DOCTOR,

With the usual melancholy I am aware that my book, which I have taken the liberty to send to you, has not fulfilled that which I had in mind. In any case, I strove with immense effort to transcend the usual feuilletonistic way of thinking.[47]

I believe that you, my dear Herr Doctor, will not share many an opinion expressed in the book; but hope very much that at the end you will regard with kindness

Your admirer
THEODOR REIK

[4]

VIENNA, 4 January 1914

MY DEAR HERR DOCTOR,

Your letter, for which I thank you very much, has given me great joy. It cannot be of any importance whether I am always right. My intention was to show the depth and breadth of your problems which the critics[48] are always trying to confine to a narrow circle.[49]

The reason for my writing, my dear Herr Doctor, is to make a request of you which I am afraid I cannot make in person. I am trying in vain for a position of any kind. This Bohemian kind of life that has been forced on me torments me as much as the miserable financial condition in which I find myself as a consequence. I would be eternally grateful to you, my dear Herr Doctor, if you would put in a good word for me with one of your influential friends. Of course I would prefer a position as an editor, a dramatic advisor, or a secretary, but I would also agree to any other type of work, as long as I could make a living from it.

It would cost you, my dear Herr Doctor, perhaps only one word to pull me out of all my misery and obtain a secure position for me.

Perhaps this thought may serve me as an insufficient excuse for my troubling you.

With great respect
Your
THEODOR REIK

[5]

BERLIN, 17 June 1914

DEAR HERR DOCTOR,

I am taking the liberty once more of contacting you again; please forgive me for doing this in the form of a request. The *Morgen* is supposed to be changed into a daily paper, as you, dear Herr Doctor, are surely aware of, and I have some hope of being given a position on its editorial staff (perhaps as a theater critic).[50] I recalled your kind promise to recommend me when the occasion arose. Perhaps, dear Herr Doctor, you know the editors of the *Morgen,* Dr. Schreier and Dr. Leoster. I would ask you kindly to recommend me to them; I know that one word from you would suffice to provide me with a livelihood. Perhaps I may appeal to your compassion; I exist under dreadful circumstances, live from hand to mouth with indescribable effort, and yet I believe myself to be fairly intelligent and useful. I would be forever obliged to you, my dear Herr Doctor, if you could do me this favor, which is of such great importance to me. I am living—only temporarily, I hope—at Berlin W.57. Bülowstrasse 24 III.

With great respect
Your grateful and devoted
THEODOR REIK

[6]

BERLIN, 20 June 1914

MY DEAR HERR DOCTOR,

I knew that you, dear Herr Doctor, would not let me plead with you in vain, and I thank you from the bottom of my heart for your kindness. An editorial position on the *Morgen* is involved. To be sure, I would prefer the feuilleton section and theater criticism, but I would agree to any type of work in the editorial office as long as it suffices to fill my small needs. At the moment I do not know what Dr. Leoster has in mind for me, but he has serious intentions of hiring me. Your very valuable recommendation will surely turn this intention into a decision.

Once more, dear Herr Doctor, I thank you with all my heart.

Most respectfully
Your admirer
THEODOR REIK

[7]

BERLIN, 7 September 1914

MY DEAR HERR DOCTOR,

With most heartfelt thanks for your good wishes, which gave much joy to my wife and me, I take the liberty to send you a small article from the *Berliner Tageblatt*.[51]

I am sure, my dear Herr Doctor, that you will remember me if you should happen to hear of any position which would be suitable for me, and I should be most grateful to you if you would then put in a good word about me. I am trying very hard to exercise "more self-control," yet I feel that this will become impossible for me in the not too distant future.

Most respectfully
Your old admirer
THEODOR REIK

[8]

BERLIN, 15 September 1914

GREATLY ESTEEMED HERR DOCTOR,

Thank you most heartily for your note which I found very

gratifying. If my article could contribute something to making people even in our old Austria think of your writings (which I love so much) in a different way, it would give me great joy. Some of your problems so greatly concern me in my own life that I am constantly occupied with them.[52]

My deeply felt gratitude, dear Herr Doctor, for your great kindness in my affairs. I would be satisfied with any position, including a "dependent" one, though I would, of course, prefer a job as editor, secretary, reader in a publishing house, etc. The *Morgen* might perhaps—one cannot be too careful when it comes to Austrian matters—be turned into a daily newspaper in the coming year. I am positive that your words on my behalf would then be of great usefulness to me.

My wife (who, incidentally, is one of your most ardent admirers) and I have rented a furnished room here and live under the narrowest and most oppressive circumstances imaginable. Therefore, I would like to take advantage of your great kindness without having too many scruples about it. If you, my dear Herr Doctor, would be so kind as to help me over the next two weeks, I believe I might be able to face the future with more security and hope. I know that you, my dear Herr Doctor, will not take my honesty the wrong way, and I am thankful to you for this as for so many other favors.

Please forgive me for troubling you with such uninteresting matters, and please retain those friendly feelings toward me which make me so very happy.

With great respect
Your devoted
THEODOR REIK

[*9*]

VIENNA, 13 October 1915

MY DEAR HERR DOCTOR,

My heartiest thanks for the kind gift of your *Comedy of Words*,[53] which, having the old force, of course is a tragicomedy of human relationships.[54]

Please forgive my not writing for such a long time (even though I felt a need for it several times): military service causes one to degenerate completely, and becomes more and more a colossal, noisy waste of time.[55]

Best regards to your wife.

With great respect
Very devotedly yours
THEODOR REIK

[*Postcard*]

[*10*]

SW Front, 18 May 1916[56]

DEAR HERR DOCTOR,

Your kind postal card, for which I thank you very much, was delayed because I was transferred and had a new address. I am under great strain. I am very homesick for my wife and child. Who knows when I will see them again—if I will see them again? I am on horseback for half days at a time. Would you, my dear Herr Doctor, continue to think of me in a friendly way? *The Road to the Open*[57] and *The Count of Charolais*[58] are the only books I have with me.

In sincere devotion
THEODOR REIK

P.S. Please remember me to your wife.

[*Postcard*]

[*11*]

22 July 1916

DEAR HERR DOCTOR,

Kindest regards from southwest front. I will take the liberty to visit you during my October furlough.

Very respectfully
THEODOR REIK

[*Postcard*]

[*12*]

Fp. 632, 27 June 1918[59]

DEAR HERR DOCTOR,

My wife sent me your kind note, for which I thank you very

much. Around the time I would have liked to come to see you, we were all [caught up] in the heaviest artillery barrage on that damned Mt. Asaloni, from where we have just returned with five wounded. When your new book is published, please do not forget

Your very devoted
THEODOR REIK

[*13*]

11 December 1918

DEAR HERR DOCTOR,

Many thanks for the gift of *Casanova's Homecoming*[60] which I have read for the second time with great enjoyment, especially as concerns the style.

In the meantime, I was successful in finding a position as political editor of the Vienna *Zeit*.[61] Please extend my best regards to your wife.

Respectfully yours
THEODOR REIK

[*14*]

VIENNA, 6 April 1922

DEAR HERR DOCTOR,

Dutch friends have written to me that you are going to Holland for some time. One of them, J. W. van Ophuijsen in The Hague, a physician in his forties, and his wife, both very nice and intelligent people who know and love your work, asked me to inquire of you if an invitation would not displease you.[62] They do not doubt that you receive too many invitations of this kind, but they would be very happy to see you and put their house and (beautiful) garden at your disposal, should you desire to have a rest. Dr. J. W. van Ophuijsen lives at The Hague, Prince Vinkenpark 5. May I answer him as to where he can send his invitation? I hope you are well, and that your stay in Holland will be rewarding and enjoyable.

With best regards
Your
THEODOR REIK

[*15*]

REICHENAU, 3 July 1923

MY DEAR HERR DOCTOR,

I was very happy about your friendly letter which was forwarded to me only now. They came on a day when I had just been reminded of your books once more, as so often happens: a patient, an American lady, spoke about you with great admiration. I am happy that my small analytical attempt stirred your interest and somewhat ashamed when I consider how inadequate and unsuitable my book about you was.[63] Perhaps I can improve it in the second edition.[64]

I would be very happy to see you again; we will return to Vienna in September. Perhaps I may be permitted to phone you then and to call on you for a walk. Or will you by chance come to Edlach during the summer? After some back and forth we finally landed in Reichenau.

With best wishes for the summer
and kind regards
Respectfully yours
THEODOR REIK

[*Calling card*]

[*16*]

[VIENNA,] 1 April 1924

DEAR HERR DOCTOR,

Many thanks for the Specht book.[65] I am ashamed that I did not send it sooner. Best regards.

Respectfully yours
THEODOR REIK

[*17*]

VIENNA, 11 December 1925

DEAR HERR DOCTOR,

Thank you very much for kindly sending me your new novella,[66] which I liked very much. The tranquil language as well as the philosophy implicit in it made a great impression on me.

By chance I received a periodical in which there is an article that might interest you; I am herewith enclosing it.

With best regards
Your
THEODOR REIK

[*18*]

VIENNA, 28 December 1927

DEAR HERR DOCTOR,

My most heartfelt thanks for your beautiful *Book of Aphorisms and Reflections*[67] which I have read slowly and with great intellectual and aesthetic pleasure. I do not agree in any way that one recognizes in each of these aphorisms thoughts and feelings of one's own. With most of these aphorisms, at least in my case, it took fairly long to recognize the truths contained within them. Perhaps it is precisely the most important truths to which we at first put up such a primary opposition.[68]

Heartiest New Year greetings and regards

Respectfully yours
THEODOR REIK

[*19*]

BERLIN, 17 November 1929

DEAR AND ESTEEMED HERR DOCTOR,

Many thanks for your kind note. I would be very happy to see you again. Please let me know in some manner when you will be in Berlin again.

In a few weeks I will take the liberty to send you a new book about Goethe in which your story *The Fate of the Baron von Leisenbohg*[69] plays a special part. You will recognize from this how much your books are in my thoughts even now.

With very best regards,

Your
THEODOR REIK

NOTES

1. A. Bronson Feldman, "Reik and the Interpretation of Literature," in *Explorations in Psychoanalysis: A Tribute to the Work of Theodor Reik,* ed. Robert Lindner (New York: Julian Press, 1953), p. 100.

2. Theodor Reik, *Fragment of a Great Confession: A Psychoanalytic Autobiography* (New York: Citadel Press, 1949), p. 25.
3. See, for example, Theodor Reik, "Arthur Schnitzler vor dem 'Anatol': Psychoanalytisches," *Pan,* 2, xxxii (June 27, 1921), 899-905; "Der kleine Anti-Schnitzler," *Pan,* 2 (1912), 1118; "Das Geschlechterverhältnis bei Arthur Schnitzler," *Neue Generation,* 9, iii (March 14, 1913), 128-135; "Schnitzler als Psycholog," *Die Persönlichkeit,* 1, iv (April, 1914), 312-313; "Arthur Schnitzler und der Krieg," *Berliner Tageblatt,* Nr. 36 (September 7, 1914). See also Theodor Reik, review of *Frau Beate und ihr Sohn,* by Arthur Schnitzler, *Imago,* 3, vi (December, 1914), 537-539. English translation: *Beatrice,* transl. Agnes Jacques (New York: AMS Press, 1971). (Reprint of 1926 edition, Simon & Schuster.) Also translated as *Mother and Son* in *Games with Love and Death* (New York: Penguin Books, 1974), pp. 9-79.
4. The original read: "Meinem verehrten Lehrer Professor Dr. Sigmund Freud in Dankbarkeit gewidmet." On January 1, 1914, Freud wrote to Reik: "All my work of the last weeks and my departure immediately afterward have made me put off answering your letter and expressing my thanks for the dedication of your fine book." Theodor Reik, *The Search Within: The Inner Experiences of a Psychoanalyst,* introd. Murray H. Sherman (New York: Jason Aronson, 1974), p. 633.
5. Theodor Reik, *The Need To Be Loved* (New York: Bantam Books, 1964), p. 57.
6. *Loc. cit.*
7. Reik, *Fragment of a Great Confession,* p. 427.
8. See, for example, Reik, *Fragment of a Great Confession,* pp. 16, 25, 184-187, 304-306, 342-344, 349, 426-430, 434-439, 442-445, 471; see also his *Jewish Wit* (New York: Gamut Press, 1962), pp. 55, 58-59, 100-101, 230, 239; *Voices from the Inaudible: The Patients Speak* (New York: Farrar, Straus and Company, 1964), pp. 10, 143-144; *Listening with the Third Ear* (New York: Pyramid Books, 1964), pp. 38-43, 102, 173; *The Need To Be Loved,* pp. 29, 55-57; *Of Lust and Love: On the Psychoanalysis of Romantic and Sexual Emotions,* introd. Murray H. Sherman (New York: Jason Aronson, 1974), pp. 174, 426, 515, 531; *The Search Within: The Inner Experiences of a Psychoanalyst,* pp. 105, 117 (pp. 87 = 16 in *Fragment,* 95 = 25 in *Fragment,* 216-219 = 426-430 in *Fragment,* 222-226 = 434-439 in *Fragment,* 274-180 = 38-43 in *Listening with the Third Ear*).
9. Reik, *Fragment of a Great Confession,* pp. 184-187.
10. Cf. Freud's letter to Schnitzler of May 14, 1922, in "Sigmund Freud: Briefe an Arthur Schnitzler," ed. Henry Schnitzler, *Neue Rundschau,* 66, i (1955), 96. (English translation in Ernst L. Freud, ed., *Letters of Sigmund Freud,* transl. Tania and James Stern [New York: Basic Books, 1960], pp. 339-340.) See also Frederick J. Beharriell, "Freud's 'Double': Arthur Schnitzler," *Journal of the American Psychoanalytic Association,* 10, i (1962), 722-730; Mark Kanzer, "Freud and His Literary Doubles," *American Imago,* 33, iii (1976), 231-243.
11. Murray H. Sherman, "Freud, Reik and the Problem of Technique in Psychoanalysis," *Psychoanalytic Review,* 52, iii (1965), 363, n. 14. English translation of Arthur Schnitzler, *The Murderer,* in *Little Novels,* transl. Eric Sutton (New York: AMS Press, 1974), pp. 221-225. (Reprint of 1929 edition.) Also translated as *The Man of Honour,* in *Games with Love and Death,* pp. 81-101.
12. Theodor Reik, Statement to Erika Freeman. In Erika Freeman, *Insights: Conversations with Theodor Reik* (Englewood Cliffs: Prentice-Hall, 1971), p. 90.
13. Anna Freud, Letter of July 11, 1971, to Jeffrey B. Berlin. Quoted with permission of Anna Freud. The original read: "Was mein Vater mit dem

'Doppelgänger' meinte, ist nicht schwer zu sagen. Er hat oft davon gesprochen, dass Dichter und Schriftsteller auf dem ihnen eigenen Weg zu denselben Schlüssen über die menschliche Natur kommen, die er mühsam in der analytischen Arbeit an Patienten erkämpfen musste. In diesem Sinn ist also der Novellist der Doppelgänger des Analytikers."

14. Bernd Urban, "Vier unveröffentlichte Briefe Arthur Schnitzlers an den Psychoanalytiker Theodor Reik," *Modern Austrian Literature,* 8, iii/iv (1975), 236-247. Urban published four of ten existent Schnitzler letters to Reik, all of which are deposited at the Houghton Library at Harvard University. The six letters left unpublished are greeting notes and provide no additional information about their relationship. We are appreciative to Bernd Urban for this information. The published letters are dated September 14, 1912; May 25, 1913; December 10, 1913; and December 31, 1913.
15. Theodor Reik, *Voices from the Inaudible: The Patients Speak,* p. 144.
16. Reik, *Listening with the Third Ear,* pp. 38-39.
17. Feldman, "Reik and the Interpretation of Literature," p. 100.
18. Robert O. Weiss, "A Study of Arthur Schnitzler with Special Consideration of the Problem of Psychosis in *Flight into Darkness,*" dissertation, Stanford University (1955), p. 48.
19. Weiss, for example, believes that "a valid psychoanalysis, like surgery, cannot be carried out on a fictitious patient. Certain interesting speculations can be made, to be sure, and even some shrewd guesses, but a person that exists only on paper cannot respond to stimuli or answer questions. This precludes *a priori* a vital part of the essential diagnostic procedure." *Ibid.,* p. 46.
20. Arthur Schnitzler, "Brief an Dr. Hans Henning," ed. Heinrich Schnitzler, *Neue Rundschau,* 68 (1957), 95-96 (our translation).
21. Reik's compulsion to read all of Gothe's works after the death of his father is well known. Reik wrote: "After the death of my father [in 1906, when Reik was eighteen] I found myself compelled by an invisible power to study and work with all my energy . . . I only know that there was suddenly the inner command to read everything that Goethe had ever written . . . I had also at this time become interested in the works of Dostoyevsky, Nietzsche, Hauptmann, and Schnitzler." Reik, *Fragment of a Great Confession,* pp. 15-16. In the section entitled "Memories of pre-Hitler Vienna" of his *Voices from the Inaudible: The Patients Speak* (p. 143), Reik observes: "One day, contrary to habit, I looked at the pictures in the vestibule of my apartment before I left it. There are some photographs of the men who were important to me when I was a student—pictures of Dostoyevsky and Schopenhauer, of Gustav Mahler and Anatole France, of Beer-Hofmann and Arthur Schnitzler."
22. Information from the records of the International Arthur Schnitzler Research Association at the State University of New York at Binghamton. Effective July, 1977, the society is located at the University of California at Riverside.
23. Mrs. Lens, Richard Beer-Hofmann's daughter, informed this writer (J.B.B.) in an interview that Reik often visited her father.
24. The term "Jung-Wien" is generally applied to the group of writers who met at the Café Griensteidl in Vienna at the turn of the century. The group mainly consisted of Raoul Auernheimer, Hermann Bahr, Richard Beer-Hofmann, Hugo von Hofmannsthal, Felix Salten, and Arthur Schnitzler. For a stimulating and profound account of this period, see Alfred Schick, "The Vienna of Sigmund Freud," *Psychoanalytic Review,* 55, iv (1968-1969), 529-551. For bibliographical information about Arthur Schnitzler, see Jeffrey B. Berlin, "Arthur Schnitzler: A Bibliography," *Modern Austrian Literature,* 4, iv (1971), 7-20; and, 6, i/ii (1973), 81-122; 7, i/ii (1974), 174-191; 8, iii/iv (1975), 248-265; 9, ii (1976), 63-72. The bibliographies are combined

in my (J.B.B.) forthcoming book on Schnitzler to be published by the Wilhelm Fink Verlag (Munich, West Germany) in January, 1978.

25. Upon Beer-Hofmann's death, Theodor Reik wrote to Mrs. Lens, Beer-Hofmann's daughter: "The news was very painful to me. Like everyone else who knew him, I loved your father. Please would you convey also to your sister and brother my expression of deep sympathy." Letter of September 27, 1945 (our translation). Reik had always sent Beer-Hofmann his books with short inscriptions, which are now in Mrs. Lens' archive. He continued to do so after Beer-Hofmann's death, as the following letter of October 3, 1949, to Mrs. Lens indicates: "I am afraid that the enclosed book will not be of great interest to you, since it belongs in the domain of scientific psychology. I am sending it to you and your sister because it contains some recollections about your father on pages 470 and 471. You know that I admired him very much. I am not satisfied with the translation of the lines from the poem *Der einsame Weg,* but perhaps it will encourage a poet to do a better job" (our translation). *Der einsame Weg* is a poem Beer-Hofmann wrote in 1905; it was dedicated to Arthur Schnitzler. *Der einsame Weg* is also the title of a Schnitzler drama. Reik offers a translation of the poem in *Fragment of a Great Confession,* p. 471. In *Voices from the Inaudible: The Patients Speak* (p. 145) Reik comments that Beer-Hofmann, who had given him a copy of the poem, had inscribed it: "For Theodor Reik in memory of past days, and most cordially."
26. Unlike Schnitzler, who kept a diary from 1879 to 1931 (that is still unpublished—although Urban cites some entries relating to Reik and Schnitzler), neither Reik nor Beer-Hofmann kept a daily record of their lives.
27. In *Voices from the Inaudible: The Patients Speak* (p. 144) Reik claims that Beer-Hofmann "was one of Schnitzler's best friends." To date little critical attention has been given to the relationship between Schnitzler and Beer-Hofmann. The most comprehensive examination remains that by Eugene Weber, "The Correspondence of Arthur Schnitzler and Richard Beer-Hofmann," *Modern Austrian Literature,* 6, iii/iv (1973), 40-51.
28. See above, n. 23.
29. Theodor Reik, *Richard Beer-Hofmann* (Leipzig: Sphinx, 1912).
30. Reik includes Sol Liptzin's translation of the *Schlaflied für Miriam* [*Lullaby for Miriam*] in chapter nineteen of *The Secret Self.* As Sol Liptzin indicated in a letter of June 24, 1975 to Murray H. Sherman, Reik made several errors in the reprinting of his translation. Possibly these errors are significant clues to Reik's personality. Harry Zohn, for one, informed us that he had written Reik about some translation errors in his book, but that "the subsequent reprints or paperback editions always had the same errors and other slips." For another poet's attitude toward the *Schlaflied für Miriam,* as well as another translation and additional information about Beer-Hofmann, see Klaus W. Jonas, "Richard Beer-Hofmann and Rainer Maria Rilke," *Modern Austrian Literature,* 8, iii/iv (1975), 43-73. When Reik sent his first book to Beer-Hofmann, he included a brief note (cf. n. 32). It is interesting to further observe that in 1913, when a conference was to be held about Beer-Hofmann, Reik first requested Beer-Hofmann's permission to speak about him. Beer-Hofmann was surprised about such a conference and neither approved nor disapproved. As this letter of May 3, 1913, then indicates, Beer-Hofmann actually was pleased that Reik would be a speaker. Beer-Hofmann further states: "You mention also the little brochure about me that you sent me some time ago. At that time I confined myself to thanking you for sending it to me and also for your kind lines that accompanied it, without seeing it as an occasion to become acquainted with you personally—something that might perhaps have seemed logical since we live in the same city. I believed—and still believe—that it is proper for a writer to keep *behind* his works. And modestly—or arrogantly, if you will—I have always declined to accept

for myself personally that which was intended for my work." He then invited Reik to visit him and expressed that he would be happy to see him. The original reads: "Sie erwähnen auch der kleinen Brochure über mich, die Sie mir seinerzeit zusandten. Ich beschränkte mich damals darauf Ihnen kurz die Zusendung und Ihre freundlichen Begleitzeilen zu danken, ohne darin—was vielleicht, da wir dieselbe Stadt bewohnen nahe lag—den Anlass zu sehen, Sie persönlich kennen zu lernen. Ich fand—und finde noch—dass es dem Dichter geziehmt, *hinter* seinem Werke zu stehen. Und, bescheiden—oder hochmütig, wenn Sie wollen—habe ich seit jeher es abgelehnt, für meine Person in Anspruch zu nehmen, was meinem Werke galt."

31. Reik, *Fragment of a Great Confession,* p. 470. Cf. below nn. 35 and 37 for Reik's further comments on the *Graf von Charolais.* Reik also briefly discusses this drama in *Jewish Wit,* pp. 69-74. To date no published English translation of the *Graf von Charolais* (Berlin: S. Fischer, 1905) exists. Among Beer-Hofmann's posthumous papers that are in the Houghton Library at Harvard University there is, however, a typewritten translation.
32. All the letters by Reik to Beer-Hofmann are handwritten and in German. The translations here are ours.
33. The original read: "Wie versprochen sende ich Ihnen heute den Abschnitt aus meiner Arbeit über Schnitzler. Ich glaube nicht, dass darin ein Zusammenhang erzwungen wird, sondern eher, dass ein zwingender Zusammenhang dargestellt wird. Wenn dies ein Verdienst ist, so gebührt der Hauptteil der Psychoanalyse." Exact certainty cannot be given to the word "June" in the date, which, in the original, appears almost illegible.
34. Letter of January 9, 1934.
35. Finally, in a letter dated July 9, 1945, Reik writes to Beer-Hofmann: "During my vacation I am working on another book in which I would like to cite the stanzas of the Präsident from the second act of *Charolais* ('Fear for the future of Desiree'). Is there a good English translation or do you know someone with sufficient poetic talent who would be prepared to translate this fairly long passage for me?" In *Listening with the Third Ear* (pp. 98-102) Reik translates the passage himself, indicating in a footnote: "The translation attempted here gives only an inadequate idea of the power, music and beauty of the original. Beer-Hofmann gave me permission to quote this passage of his play."
36. See pp. 173-177 and *The Need To Be Loved,* pp. 229-230.
37. The original read: "Vielen Dank für Ihre freundliche Karte, die ich infolge Abkommandierung und neuer Feldpostadresse verspätet erhielt. Bin fast den ganzen Tag im Sattel. Würde mich sehr freuen, wenn Sie mir erlaubten Sie wieder zu besuchen, wenn ich zurückkomme—*wenn ich* zurückkomme. Der 'Graf von Charolais,' den ich mithabe, hat mir in diesen Tagen etwas wie Trost und Beruhigung gebracht wie schon oft."
38. The original read: "Lese eben in der Zeitung, dass wir den "Grafen von Charolais" nun wohl für immer auch in Wien haben werden und freue mich darüber. Hier erlebt man manchmal so Grauenhaftes, dass man glaubt, man werde nie mehr im Leben lachen können."
39. Reik, *Fragment of a Great Confession,* p. 471.
40. Urban, "Vier unveröffentlichte Briefe Arthur Schnitzlers an den Psychoanalytiker Theodor Reik," 241.
41. *Ibid.,* p. 242.
42. With the exception of letter 17, which is typed, all are handwritten. All the originals are in German, which we have translated.
43. Theodor Reik, *Arthur Schnitzler als Psycholog* (Minden: J. C. Bruns, 1913). Cf. the reviews of the book: Max Koch in *Die schöne Literatur,* 15, x (May 9, 1914), 185-186; Josef Körner in *Das Literarische Echo,* 19, xiii (April, 1917), 802-805; Hanns Sachs in *Imago,* 3 (1914), 302-304.

44. Theodor Reik, *Flaubert und seine "Versuchung des Heiligen Antonius": Ein Beitrag zur Künstlerpsychologie* (Minden: J. C. Bruns, 1912).
45. See above, n. 4.
46. The original read: "Ich erlaube mir, anzufragen, ob ich et Ihnen, sehr geehrter Herr Doktor, widmen darf. Ihre Erlaubnis würde mich sehr freuen."
47. The original read: "Ich bin mir mit der üblichen Wehmut bewusst, dass mein Buch, das ich mir erlaube, Ihnen zu senden, nicht das, was mir vorschwebte, erfüht hat. Immerhin habe ich mit heissem Bemühen darnach gestrebt, über die gewöhnliche feuilletonistische Betrachtungsweise hinauszukommen. Ich glaube, dass Sie, sehr verehrter Herr Doktor, manche Ansicht des Buches nicht teilen werden; hoffe aber sehr, dass Sie am Ende in Freundlichkeit gedenken Ihres Sie verehrenden Theodor Reik." Cf. n. 33.
48. Early Schnitzler critics were very limited in their approach, as Beharriell, for one, explains: "One hears repeatedly that Schnitzler offers just one mood, just one set of characters, just one milieu; especially his 'one problem,' the psychology of frivolous love." Frederick Beharriell, "Arthur Schnitzler's Range of Theme," *Monatshefte*, 43, vii (1951), 301.
49. The original read: "Ihr Brief, für den ich bestens danke, hat mir viel Freude gemacht. Es kann nicht darauf ankommen, ob ich überall Recht habe. Meine Absicht war, die Tiefe und Weite Ihrer Probleme, welche die Kritiker in einen engen Kreis bannen wollen, zu zeigen."
50. It is unknown if Reik obtained this position.
51. S. Fischer also sent Schnitzler a copy of Reik's article. In a letter dated September 11, 1914, Schnitzler indicates to Fischer that he found Reik's essay extremely gratifying. (Schnitzler, Letter of September 11, 1914, in Peter de Mendelssohn, *S. Fischer und sein Verlag* [Frankfurt am Main: S. Fischer Verlag, 1970], p. 693.) Reik's article presents many good points; for example, he observes: "An additional fact can be discovered here by the attentive listener to and reader of Schnitzler's works: the human, or rather, the psychic necessity of the military profession. This, to be sure, concerns not the institution of militarism, which Schnitzler often subjected to unsparing criticism, but the satisfaction of the inner needs of a certain not at all rare type of individual. Felix Wegrath in *Der einsame Weg* may be included among this type . . . Another such soldier, Leutnant Karinski in *Freiwild,* Schnitzler has described by a comrade-in-arms: 'How can such a man contain his spirits during an eternal time of peace? What outlet does he have for them? There is no doubt, people like Karinski should be soldiers, but for such soldiers war is a necessity, otherwise there is no justification for their existence'" (our translation). Theodor Reik, "Arthur Schnitzler und der Krieg," *Berliner Tageblatt,* Nr. 36 (September 7, 1914). The original read: "Noch etwas kann der aufmerksame Zuhörer und Leser Schnitzlerscher Werke hier erfassen: die menschliche, will sagen seelische Notwendigkeit des Soldatenberufes. Es handelt sich, wohlgemerkt, nicht um die Institution des Militarismus, die Schnitzler oft einer unerbittlichen Kritik unterzogen hat, sondern um die Befriedigung innerer Bedürfnisse eines bestimmten, gar nicht seltenen Menschentyps. Felix Wegrath im 'Einsamen Weg' darf zu diesem Typ gerechnet werden . . . Der Oberleutnant Karinski in 'Freiwild' ist ein Mensch, der in andere Verhältnisse hineingehört. Ein Regimentskamerad schildert ihn: 'Um sich hauen musst' er können. Was fängt so ein Mensch in ewiger Friedenszeit mit seinem Temperament an? Wo soll er hin damit? Es ist ja wahr solche Leute wie der Karinski sollen Soldaten sein, aber für solche Soldaten gehört der Krieg, sonst haben sie überhaupt keine Berechtigung.'"
52. The original read: "Wenn mein Artikel dazu ein wenig beitragen konnte, dass man auch in unserem alten Österreich Ihre Werke, die ich so sehr liebe, anders betrachten lernt, würde ich mich aufrichtig freuen. Einige Ihrer

Probleme gehen mir im eigenen Leben so sehr nach, dass ich mich beständig mit ihnen beschäftigen muss." Some of Schnitzler's themes include love, death, illusion and reality, truth and lying, jealousy, loneliness, anguish, fate, and chance.

53. Arthur Schnitzler, *Komödie der Worte* (Berlin: S. Fischer, 1915). The *Komödie der Worte* is comprised of three one-act plays: *Stunde des Erkennens, Grosse Szene,* and *Das Bacchusfest.* English translation: *Comedy of Words* and *Other Plays,* transl. Pierre Loving (Cincinnati: Stewart & Kidd, 1917).
54. The original read: "Meinen herzlichsten Dank für die liebenswürdige Übersending Ihrer 'Komödie der Worte,' die, mit der alten Gewalt wirkend, doch eine Tragikomödie der menschlichen Beziehungen ist."
55. Cf. n. 36.
56. On the same day Reik wrote a similar letter to Beer-Hofmann; cf. n. 37.
57. Arthur Schnitzler, *Der Weg ins Freie* (Berlin: S. Fischer, 1908). English translation: *The Road to the Open,* transl. Horace Samuel (New York: Alfred A. Knopf, 1923).
58. See above, n. 31.
59. On this same day Reik also wrote Beer-Hofmann: "Best regards, my dear Herr Doctor, after my return from Mt. Asalone, where we spent a week under the strongest artillery fire."
60. Arthur Schnitzler, *Casanovas Heimfahrt* (Berlin: S. Fischer, 1918). English translation: *Casanova's Homecoming,* transl. Eden and Cedar Paul (New York: AMS Press, 1971). (Reprint of 1930 edition, New York: Simon & Schuster.)
61. Apparently Reik had previously requested Schnitzler's aid. On October 8, 1918, Reik wrote Beer-Hofmann: "Please forgive me if I annoy you with a request at this turbulent time for you. Dr. Schnitzler, whom I recently visited, advised me to turn to you with this request. When you get a chance, would you ask Reinhardt if he would take me on as a dramatic advisor or in a similar position after demobilization? Would you be so kind? I should be most grateful to you." Schnitzler and Max Reinhardt were not on cordial terms, and presumably this is why Schnitzler refers Reik to Beer-Hofmann (cf. *Der Briefwechsel Arthur Schnitzlers mit Max Reinhardt und dessen Mitarbeitern,* ed. Renate Wagner [Salzburg: Otto Müller Verlag, 1971]). The next month, on November 18, 1918, Reik again wrote to Beer-Hofmann: "Please forgive me for bothering you again with a request. You were kind enough to ask me to turn to you if you could be useful in my search for a position. I am now planning to find a position with the Jewish Community Council (archives, library, etc.) and in this connection I wanted to inquire if you, my dear Herr Doctor, might know someone whose influence could be of some use to me. Do you think Dr. Feuchtwang whom I recently visited and with whom I spoke about several points in the history of religion might be able to do something for me?"
62. Schnitzler traveled to Holland from April 19 to May 19, 1922, during which time he gave readings. Cf. Reinhard Urbach, *Schnitzler Kommentar zu den erzählenden Schriften und dramatischen Werken* (Munich: Winkler Verlag, 1974), p. 74. It is unknown if Schnitzler visited the Ophuijsen family. It should be noted that J. W. Ophuijsen (1882-1950), who came to New York from Holland in 1935, was a prominent psychoanalyst.
63. The original read: "Ich habe mich sehr über Ihre freundliche Zeilen, die mir erst jetzt nachgeschickt wurden, gefreut. Sie kamen gerade an einem Tage, da ich wieder wie so oft an Ihre Bücherss erinnert wurde: eine amerikanische Patientin sprach mit grosser Bewunderung von Ihnen. Ich bin froh darüber, dass mein kleiner analytischer Versuch Ihre Interesse erregt hat, und einigermassen beschämt, wenn ich daran denke, wie unzulflnglich und

unangemessen mein Buch über Sie war. Vielleicht kann ich es in der zweiten Auflage besser machen."

64. A second edition never appeared.
65. Richard Specht, *Arthur Schnitzler: Der Dichter und sein Werk, Eine Studie* (Berlin: S. Fischer Verlag, 1922). Specht is one of the few early critics whose interpretations surpassed the generalizations of his contemporaries.
66. In 1924 Schnitzler published *Fräulein Else.* Possibly this is the work, but it is more likely that Reik received *Die Frau des Richters,* which appeared in August, 1925. Cf. Urbach, *Schnitzler-Kommentar,* pp. 74-75.
67. Arthur Schnitzler, *Buch der Sprüche und Bedenken. Aphorismen und Fragmente* (Vienna: Phaidon Verlag, 1927). Now in *Aphorismen und Betrachtungen,* ed. Robert O. Weiss (Frankfurt am Main: S. Fischer Verlag, 1967). To date only one section has been translated; see Arthur Schnitzler, "Work and Echo: A Collection of Animadversions on the Artist, the Theory of Abstract Art and Dramatic Art," *Vanity Fair* (November, 1928), pp. 78, 130-132, 138. A few aphorisms were also published in 1928 in *Plain Talk.* Not all the aphorisms translated there were written by Schnitzler, even though they carry his name. This subject is discussed in greater detail in my (J.B.B.) forthcoming study of the history and development of Schnitzler's work in the United States, which is based upon Schnitzler's still unpublished letters to his publishers, agents, translators, and critics. The aphorism on the title page of Schnitzler's *Buch der Sprüche und Bedenken* is "Tiefsinn hat nie ein Ding erhellt/Klarsinn schaut tiefer in die Welt." In *Voices from the Inaudible: The Patients Speak* (pp. 143-144), Reik notes that Schnitzler had inscribed these lines on a photograph of himself that he gave Reik. (Reik uses the word *blickt* instead of Schnitzler's *schaut.*) After translating these lines as "By profound thought no thing was ever clarified/ Clear thought pervades the world with deeper light," Reik further observes: "For a moment I look again into his [Schnitzler's] steel-blue eyes and listen to his voice as I did so often on our walks in Vienna. Recently I read the commemorative speech on Schnitzler by Franz Werfel . . . who calls the poet 'master of loneliness' and contends that 'loneliness forms the essential content of all his works and characters, from the first to the last. . . .' A remark Schnitzler once made to me came to mind: 'One can feel really lonely only in company.' "
68. The original read: "Meinen herzlichen Dank für Ihr schönes 'Buch der Sprüche und Bedenken,' das ich langsam und mit grossem intellektuellen und ästhetischen Genuss gelesen habe. Ich bin keineswegs damit einverstanden, dass man in jedem dieser Sprüche Selbstgedachtes oder gefühltes erkennt. Bei den meisten hat es, zumindestens bei mir, einer längeren Zeit bedurft, um die in ihnen enthaltene Wahrheit wiederzuerkennen. Vielleicht sind es gerade die wichtigsten Wahrheiten, denen wir zuerst einen solchen primären Widerstand entgegensetzen."
69. Arthur Schnitzler, *Das Schicksal des Freiherrn von Leisenbohg,* in *Gesammelte Werke: Die Erzählenden Schriften* (Frankfurt am Main: S. Fischer Verlag, 1961). Vol. I, pp. 580-597. English translation: *The Fate of the Baron* in *Little Novels,* pp. 9-36. In 1929 Reik published in *Imago* (Vol. 15, pp. 400-537) *Warum verliess Goethe Friedericke? Eine psychoanalytische Monographie.* Schnitzler's work is discussed there, and in all probability this is the book sent to Schnitzler. Now in *Fragment of a Great Confession,* see esp. pp. 184-187.

Jeffrey B. Berlin, Dept of Humanities
Philadelphia College of Textiles and Science
School Lane and Henry Avenue
Philadelphia, Pa. 19144

SCHNITZLER AND FREUD AS DOUBLES: Poetic Intuition and Early Research on Hysteria

Bernd Urban
Translated by John Menzies and Peter Nutting

We contemporaries are mysteriously important to each other.
—Hugo von Hofmannsthal

In an often cited letter from Freud[1] to Schnitzler on Schnitzler's sixtieth birthday, Freud said he avoided the poet "out of a kind of shyness at the thought of seeing my double."[2] Freud continued,

> Not that I am easily inclined to identify[3] myself with another or that I want to disregard the difference in ability that separates me from you, but when I become absorbed in your beautiful creations I always believe I find behind the poetic appearance the presuppositions, interests, and results that are already known to me as my own.

Freud came across a work, possibly for the first time, that Schnitzler had written a quarter of a century before, and Freud was astonished "how much a creative writer knows about things."[4] Freud hardly realized at this point what sort of "presuppositions" and "interests" were hidden in this writer and easily ascribed them to that almost unlimited capacity which creative writers appeared to have, and because of which he offered the greatest reverence, even love, to them as to no other writers.[5] Through "intuition," Freud wrote further in that birthday letter, Schnitzler knew everything that

* From *Germanisch-Romanische Monatsschrift,* New Series, Vol. 24, No. 2, June 1974, pp. 193-223, and reprinted with the permission of the publisher.

0033-2836/78/1300-0131 $00.95 © 1978 N.P.A.P.

Freud "had discovered in other men after laborious work." "Intuition" he explained incisively as "really . . . the result of close self-observation."[6] The analyst has again moved dangerously close to that limit where he begins to dissolve "a piece of supposed arbitrariness (. . .) into regularity,"[7] and also to explain gifted intuition and thereby diverts easily from his own intuition, but interprets unawares the knowledge of his own psyche.

Schnitzler nominally "discovered" much psychoanalytic theory earlier than Freud and independently of him—at least so Frederick J. Baharriell demonstrated.[8] Schnitzler's work *On Functional Aphonia and Its Treatment Through Hypnosis and Suggestion* "anticipates Freud's work on hypnotism and neurosis by four years,"[9] wrote Beharriell. Could the Breuer-Freud *Studies on Hysteia* (1895) have brought new insights to the creative writer? Schnitzler's early sketch *Spring Night in the Dissection Chamber* (1880) anticipates Freud's "most valuable discovery," *The Interpretation of Dreams* (1900), and could even "claim for itself priority of discovery." The short story *The Sensitive One* (1895) presupposes the "sexual causes of hysteria." More examples could be culled from the early works of Schnitzler, and still other elements of psychoanalysis may be foreshadowed: nymphomania in *The Bride,* ambivalent feelings of a husband toward his rival in *The Other,* infantile dreams and their meaning in *The Son.* Baharriell considered the year 1894 a dividing point, because Freud's only publications till then had consisted of several translations and the essay he wrote with Breuer *On the Psychic Mechanism of Hysterial Phenomena.* Finally, Beharriell wrote,

> Without exaggeration it can be said that already prior to 1894 Schnitzler's writings show all the convictions and knowledge which in his later works were considered to have been obviously influenced by Freud.[10]

Fundamentals first. In 1923 Freud expressed an opinion on the question of "anticipation" of his theories, especially the theory of dreams. He wrote:

> There is much of interest to be said about the appearance of scientific originality. When a new idea appears in science which is appraised a discovery at first, and as such is generally opposed,

> objective research soon demonstrates that there is really no novelty. As a rule it has already been done repeatedly, often at times very far removed from one another, and then forgotten, or it has already at least had precursors, was surmised or incompletely expressed. That is too well known to require further discussion.
>
> But also the subjective side of originality is worthy of exploration. A scientific worker may well ask himself where he gets the particular ideas that he brings to his material. Then without much reflection he finds that he goes back to some of those ideas for more stimulation, ideas which he has taken up and modified in their consequences on the other hand. For another portion of his ideas he cannot find anything similar. He must suppose that these thoughts and points of view have originated in his own thought process—he does not know how. Through them he supports his claim to originality.
>
> Careful psychological investigation limits this claim still further. It uncovers hidden, long-forgotten sources from which the stimulus of the apparently original ideas flowed, and substitutes in place of the supposed new creation a revitalization of the forgotten in the application to new material. There is nothing regrettable in this. One has no right to expect that the original would be underived and undetermined. In my own case, the originality of many new ideas that I used in the interpretation of dreams and psychoanalysis evaporated.[11]

That is essentially true likewise of Freud's research on classical hysterical symptoms, because they were depicted "already hundreds of years earlier in the writings on demonic possession," documents Freud studied.[12] Alfred Freiherr von Berge, later director of the Burg-Theater in Vienna, called the whole theory advanced in Breuer and Freud's *Studies* "only a piece of age-old poetic psychology."[13,14]

When Baharriell believed he saw in Schnitzler's early works "all the principal attributes" of later psychoanalysis—

> the hidden depths of personality, the various levels of consciousness, the control of the subconscious over the conscious, doubt of free will, knowledge about the meaning of dreams, the immense influence of childhood experiences on the development and the psychological meaning of sexual impressions

—it is then to be asked which of these elements had not been accessible to poets since time immemorial and where Freud had failed to cite poets as crowning witnesses for his theories.[15]

Schnitzler too cannot be said to be wholly original, since his work grew from the tradition of poets whose "most real domains" were "the portrayal of human psychic life."[16] Freud admitted unabashedly that the poet "was always the precursor of science and also scientific psychology."

But here it is a sidetrack to analyse originality per se. Our subject requires that Freud's understanding of originality be applied to the ideas of Freud and Schnitzler, that we ask whether there are similarities in ideas between the two men, and if so whether the similarities seem coincidental and exceptional or are the result of the influence of one man on the other, and if so which on which, and what part these ideas played in the development of psychoanalysis.

Freud's view of originality contains not only the astounding admission that the "originality of many new thoughts" of *The Interpretation of Dreams* evaporated, but also an attempt to clear the last spot occupied by an autonomous idea: he relinquished the claim that he had "originally discovered dream distortion," to the poet Popper-Lynkeus,[17] who described it in his *Fantasies of a Realist.*[18]

Such a weighty and self-effacing concession was possible for the creator of psychoanalysis only to creative writers, or perhaps archaeology.[19] Freud feared his own psyche in which poetic impulses had manifested themselves early and had even—bound to philosophical speculation—begun to overflow dangerously.[20] On account of this he may have "felt, if not recognized, the necessity of an unrelenting disciplining of his thought."[21] This influenced his choice of profession.

> As is known, Freud himself has emphasized that in his own judgment he was not a "real doctor." After many years of patient laboratory work and a strict drilling in the scientific method, he returned to the subjects of his youth. "My life's triumph lies in the fact that after a great detour I found the original direction."

There is a strange similarity to Schnitzler, and still more to Schnitzler's father. The gift for creative writing that expressed itself early grew in a medical-professorial environment, but the father had already composed dramas in Hungarian and German while in secondary school. Schnitzler wrote in his autobiography *Youth in Vienna*[22] that his father had been prophesied to become the "Hungarian Shakespeare," but

> After reading the Hyrtlian anatomy,[23] which stimulated him on one school vacation, he gave up all future literary plans and decided enthusiastically upon a medical career; but he still declared up to his last years, not only to me, that according to his gifts he had been entitled to at least the same literary aspirations as I was.

That could have been true for Freud, but not the "enthusiasm" which Schnitzler's father manifested in his choice of career—neither for him nor for Arthur Schnitzler. The son's aversion to the medical profession and opposition to the monotony of his practice could not be hidden.[24] Hardly a year after his graduation in 1886, he wrote,

> I spent almost half a year as assistant doctor in the psychiatric division of Professor Meynert,[25] the so-called observation room, and had hardly been more industrious there than the service demanded. Naturally, there were cases which interested me; I conducted my case histories in a decent way, took part in the visits, read all kinds of pertinent things, but it was not a question of actual scientific work.[26]

In the same year the father founded the *Internationale Klinische Rundschau* (*International Clinical Review*), and from January of 1887 the son was its editor. But he did not feel completely at home; "the little everyday medical-journalistic tasks" which he "had to perform now more than before" brought him no joy:

> Primarily I was active as a compiler, excerpted articles that had appeared in other professional journals, summarized reports of domestic and foreign meetings, read corrections, wrote a short or long report now and then for which my father occasionally praised me, and distinguished myself on the whole in the medical-journalistic area as little as in all other areas that I had formerly entered, so I seemed more condemned than ever to run through my earthly existence as the son of my father.[27,28]

And he looked more deeply into his self-discontentment:

> If one looked into this hundred-times-scattered existence of a young doctor, poet, and bon vivant, who at worst bungled in creative

writing, medicine, and life and at best was a dilettante whose being was known by one and barely conceived of by himself—this person, surrounded by dozens of friends, none of whom he belonged to completely, and by many girls and women, none of whom belonged completely to him—this person, doubtlessly unsatisfied, not without self-seeking impulses, occupied himself exclusively with himself. Would no powerful light from outside fall onto this existence (which was inwardly so unsurely illuminated by so many flickering lamps), before which light those small lights were extinguished for a few minutes at least?[29]

Two years later he wrote:

And still, it was no longer the completely usual trot. It almost appeared that I would progress slowly, very slowly of course, now in this direction, now in that. I had begun to occupy myself with hypnotism, the interest in which had become very lively primarily through the work of Charcot[30] and Bernheim; I succeeded in treating several cases of functional aphonia, i.e., of voicelessness without demonstrable organic change in the vocal organs, by way of hypnosis or through suggestion alone, and I published the case histories relating to this in the *Internationale Klinische Rundschau.*[31]

Schnitzler then told how he, with an interest that was more than purely medical, conducted experiments in hypnotism. It was

stimulating when I let my hypnotized patient go through all sorts of situations and sensations as it pleased me to invent them. I even arranged, from one day to another, a murder attempt against myself, from which I could successfully protect myself, of course, since I was prepared for it down to the minute and it was attempted with a dull paper knife rather than with a dagger. Not only my closer colleagues in the department, but also other doctors in the clinic and from other hospitals occasionally appeared at my experiments. Those who appeared most often maliciously spread it around that I conducted "performances" at the Polyclinic, and this at first caused me to close my experiments to the general public, although I still continued them awhile longer among a smaller circle.[32] But this time too I lacked the consistency to continue in the direction I had begun, and when in addition I noticed that precisely my most interesting patients were injured by the repetition of the experiments, not only in their strength of will but also in

> their physical health, I desisted from further experiments of a purely psychological nature and applied hypnosis only in individual cases, almost exclusively for clearly defined healing purposes.

Experimentation stood near the limits of medical ethics; scientific seriousness and frivolity[33] lay close together.

Nevertheless, this description is not to be completely trusted. The poet is too biased against the medical course his young life was taking; the medical tradition in his family, as well as that with which this profession has been provided from time immemorial, induced Schnitzler, in looking back, to put himself into more discredit[34] than the soul wished to admit—the soul which projected its depth and seriousness into the figures of doctors in his literary work, unconsciously and consciously at the same time. Here lies the true stratum,[35] and here lie the correlations of the early doctor-writer phase as well as to Freud again. Freud was incomparably more serious about his scientific work. His early letters and other papers reveal an honest, straightforward, passionate scientist;[36] he observed, as well he might, how "the rabble enjoyed itself" while he and his fiancée had to be sparing of their health, enjoyment, and excitation: "We are preserving ourselves for something—for what we are not sure—and this habit of continual suppression of natural drives gives us the character of refinement," so he consoled Martha in a letter of August 29, 1883,[37] writing, as Schnitzler did a little later in his reviews of medical works,

> The poor are too powerless, too exposed, to do as we do. When I see people enjoy themselves by setting aside all discretion, then I always think that it is their compensation for all the taxes, epidemics, illnesses, and abuses of the social institutions which strike them helpless.[38]

The evasiveness of Schnitzler[39] corresponds to the habit of Freud, when he wrote, for example, as early as 1908 in the foreword to *The Interpretation of Dreams*, about the meaning his father's death had for him:

> It proved to be, as I realized during my self-analysis, . . . the most meaningful event, the most decisive loss in my life.[40]

In the foreword to the first edition he cleverly circumvented the necessity and foundations of that self-analysis—this as well a "strategy of self-concealment and self-disguise"[41]—and wrote:

> It turned out that inextricably bound up with the communication of my own dreams was the fact that I was more open to unfamiliar insights through the intimacies of my psychic life than was welcome to me, and than otherwise is the task of an author who is not a creative writer but a scientist. That was painful but unavoidable. Therefore I acquiesced in this in order not to have to renounce the authenticity of my psychological results. Naturally, I could still not resist the temptation to blunt the point through exclusions and replacements of some indiscretions; as often as this happened, it contributed to the value of the examples used by me in the most decisively disadvantageous way.[42]

Thus *The Interpretation of Dreams* itself could be subjected to "pathographic" interpretation,[43] as it is practiced on some literary works, even Schnitzler's.[44] Those neurotic disturbances that threatened to take the upper hand in the middle of Freud's manhood and gave a measure of intensity to his work on the interpreting of dreams[45] were masterfully overplayed by him, shunted to others, diverting suspicion:

> I had to choose between my own dreams and those of my patients in psychoanalytic treatment. Patients' dreams were less useful because the events in them were subject to an undesirable complication due to the intervention of the patients' neurotic characteristics.[46]

The correspondence of his youth and letters to his fiancée[47] already showed intensive self-observation, "not only from an interest in psychic phenomena, which was no doubt originally present, but, much more, because his own neurotic disturbances drove him to it."[48] Something like this may likewise have motivated Schnitzler to begin his diary, for he wrote on August 10, 1890: "I have a special need to hold onto myself psychologically. Why? In order to bring a bit of peace into my tormented nervous system? From egotism? From literary interest?"[49]

Werfel's commemorative words on Schnitzler after Schnitzler's death are true of Freud as well: "He was so very incorruptible that he could not even corrupt himself. The battleground of his life lay not in the outside world, but in his conscience."[50]

Schnitzler's joyless medical activity, the medical contributions that he wrote without pleasure, his lack of perseverance in scientific activity—all this he expressed even in his medical works, which speak in their own weighty tone, even those which were printed in professional journals before the turn of the century.[51] Here we also come across the first dates.

In Schnitzler's early medical papers and reviews Freud's name first appears at the end of 1886 in a small discussion[52] of Charcot's *New Lectures on the Diseases of the Nervous System, Especially on Hysteria,* which were published in the same year in Freud's translation. Only a few weeks later at the beginning of 1887 a detailed review by Schnitzler of the work appeared in the *Internationale Klinische Rundschau.*[53] In this review Schnitzler began to speak of a lecture that Freud delivered in 1886. Freud lectured to the Society of Doctors on two themes: *On Male Hysteria*[54] and *Toward the Causality of Hysteria,*[55] the latter shortly before the end of the year. Schnitzler went into this: "When Dr. Freud recently brought up the theme in the Royal Imperial Society of Doctors in Vienna," there developed "a lively discussion."[56] Freud wrote similarly in his *Self-Portrait.*[57] The first lecture, on the other hand, summarized the results of Freud's study of Charcot but led to a discussion with Meynert, probably because Freud had "implicitly" drawn attention "to the failings of the Viennese Medical School."[58] Schnitzler, in any case, agreed with Freud's oral summary in his review when he discussed the waivering concept of neurosis, the phenomena of male hysteria, and hysterical paralyses in Charcot's work. In the review of 1886 Schnitzler had already praised the "outstanding translation by Dr. Freud" which followed closely on "all the earlier works of the trustworthy neuropathologist,"[59] and he now wrote:

> Dr. Freud has translated the book in such an outstanding way that one is hardly anywhere reminded that one has a translation before him. He has enriched German literature with a new work, earning the gratitude of German doctors and the recognition of the critics in equal measure.[60]

Schnitzler praised the translator again one year after the book's appearance (189) in the discussion of Bernheim's *Suggestion and Its Healing Power,*[61] and still later in the 1892 reviews of Bernheim's *New Studies on Hypnotism, Suggestion, and Psychotherapy* and Charcot's *Polyclinical Lectures.*[62] These are the main works on hysteria, hypnosis, and suggestion in which Freud was authoritatively involved. Schnitzler referred to Bernheim's *Suggestion and Its Healing Power* in his *Aphonia* study of 1889.[63] Mitchell's book, *The Treatment of Certain Forms of Neurasthenia and Hysteria,* appeared before that; both Schnitzler and Freud reviewed it.[64] Finally, Schnitzler was struck by Freud's research on cocaine,[65] as verified by his review of Erlenmeyer's[66] *Morphine Addiction and Its Treatment,*[67] one of Schnitzler's first major discussions that went beyond medical problems. The social ramifications of addiction were discussed,[68] and Schnitzler noted:

> A book could be written about that alone which would certainly not lack cultural-historical interest. Nor could a philanthropist refrain from a slight shudder at hearing of the strange Parisian fashion according to which the ladies of certain social circles wear morphine syringes on their watch chains as elegant trinkets. Does this not echo the peculiarity we perceive in the highly developed acquisitive sense of some pharmacists and druggists who forget to wait for the prescriptions of the doctor? Will we not be tempted to explain many a strange event with our insight that in morphine lies the dangerous power to corrupt characters, to change the respectable, reliable man into an ethical invalid? And finally, the officer addicted to morphine who falls asleep on his horse, the lawyer who must be awakened before the plea—are they not characteristic episodic figures in this strange and multifaceted picture?
>
> Thus the study of morphine addiction which takes on a meaning, which goes far beyond a professional desire for knowledge and an abundance of energetic details, continually leads us to the old adage that the doctor should not merely be a doctor of medicine, but much more.[69]

At times there lay a danger here, for the accusation was made that the influence of those doctors who were hypnotizing and using suggestion bordered on charlatanry. In the very year when Schnitzler reported on his own hypnosis experiments in his *Aphonia* study, and added the hypnosis scene[70] to his cycle *Anatol* in *The Question to Destiny,*[71] Freud had to defend in a seven-column review Forel's *Hypnotism, Its Meaning and Management* (1889):

> The attacks of the opponents, strangely enough, are in no way aimed at suggestion. The use of suggestion is ostensibly something which is familiar to the doctor at all times. "We are all constantly using suggestion," so they say. And in fact the doctor, even the nonhypnotist, is never more satisfied than when he has repressed a symptom of disease from the attention of a patient through the power of his personality, through the influence of his speech and authority. Why shouldn't the doctor, therefore, methodically strive for an influence which is ever after desirable to him if he succeeds in it once unexpectedly? Is not suggestion perhaps reproachable, the suppression of the free personality through the doctor who maintains direction over the sleeping brain even in artificial sleep? It is very interesting to see the most decided determinists suddenly become defenders of the endangered "personal freedom of will"[72]—such as the psychiatrist who is used to suffocating the "free striving intellectual activity" of his patients with large doses of bromine, morphine, and chloral—it is interesting to hear the influence of suggestion attacked as demeaning for both parties. Can one really forget that the suppression of the independence of the patient through hypnotic suggestion is always only partial, that it is directed against the symptoms of disease? It has been demonstrated hundreds of times that the entire social education of man rests on a suppression of useless ideas, concepts and motives and their replacement by better ones; that everyday life brings to every man psychic impressions, which although they intrude into the waking state, change him far more extensively than the suggestion of the doctor who seeks to remove an idea of pain or anxiety through an effective counter-idea. No, there is nothing dangerous in hypnotic therapy unless it is misused, and whatever doctor is not capable of the care or purity of intention necessary to avoid this misuse would do well to stay far away from this new method of treatment.[73]

Just a few years later Freud described the role of the doctor during the treatment of hysteria:

> With others who have agreed to give themselves over to the doctor and give him some trust, something they do voluntarily, never through coercion—with these others, I say, it is hardly to be avoided that the personal relationship to the doctor does not force itself into the foreground improperly for a while; it even seems as if such an intrusion of the doctor is the condition solely under which the solution of the problem is permitted.[74]

Here lie Freud's basic experiences of "resistance" and "transference" within psychoanalytic treatment[75] to which he later dedicated corrective explanations again and again. At the same time in the chapter "On the Psychotherapy of Hysteria" in *Studies on Hysteria,* those basic concepts of psychoanalytic theory are described which later brought Freud so much hostility: the concept of psychic determination, the function of neurotic symptoms,[76] the practice of free association, which encouraged the patient to uncritically communicate whatever came into his mind, delivered the patient into the hands of the doctor, even in his waking state.[77] This is relevant here inasmuch as Freud began as early in 1890 to turn away from the relatively unreliable hypnotic technique in order to develop—after experiments with the "pressure-procedure"—that free association technique which he began to use around 1892 with such patients as Elisabeth von R.[78]

Schnitzler had come across the same difficulties. "In no way would I want to omit hypnosis and suggestion from among the therapeutic implements that I take to the field against functional illnesses," he wrote at the end of his work *On Functional Aphonia and Its Treatment Through Hypnosis and Suggestion,*[79] but he admitted that several of the hypnosis experiments he undertook miscarried, and that the cases had by no means safe prognosis:

> Thus I would not dare to place the bold word "healed" under one of my cases, although at the moment these lines are written, most all the patients appear to have been favorably influenced in their functional aphonia through suggestive treatment.

The flaws lay in the nature of hypnosis: with some patients it did not work or the power of suggestion was only briefly effective. While Schnitzler did not investigate this further, Freud fully developed the "technical assistance of hypnosis" and refined the method of free association, a procedure he distinguished from the actual psychoanalytical procedure. This he impressively described in the chapter "On the Psychotherapy of Hysteria" at the end of the *Studies on Hysteria.*[80]

The "break with previous development"[81] lets us go back to the beginning of the eighties when Josef Breuer[82] began to treat Anna O.[83] and came to know Freud. Freud followed the progress of the case with great interest and wrote in retrospect:

> The girl became ill from the care of her dearly loved father. Breuer could now prove that all her symptoms were related to this nursing and found their explanation through it.[84]

In the course of the treatment, which covered many years, Breuer observed how damaging had been the influence of intensive, effectively inhibiting nursing, and he pointed out the etiological significance of "hypnoid states":

> Nursing produces—through stillness, the concentration on an object, and listening to the breathing of the patient—the very same conditions as many methods of hypnosis and fills the twilight state that originates in this way with anxiety.[85]

With that patient, Breuer discovered the cathartic method—Breuer and Freud took over her "talking cure" and "chimney-sweeping."[86] Traumatic affects were unleashed in the hypnotic state. In this case both predecessors of psychoanalysis, hypnosis and the cathartic method, were discussed. Freud wrote, "Theoretically as well as therapeutically, a new method governs psychoanalysis which has emerged from hypnotism," and, "The cathartic method is the immediate predecessor of psychoanalysis, and despite all expansions of experience and all modifications of the theory it is still its core.[87]

Freud was already at work when in 1885 Schnitzler received his doctorate in medicine; Freud had already encountered the characteristic hysterial symptoms of aphasia and aphonia in the same year in his work with Charcot. And he treated aphasia in a critical study in 1891 (of course dealing with the nuerological aspects), two years after Schnitzler's work on aphonia; but in 1888 he had described those signs of aphasia and aphonia as characteristic of the symptomatology of hysteria in a thirteen-column lexicon article entitled "Hysteria."[88] Moreover, he had dealt with aphasia in a separate article. Time and again, since 1885, he had been impressed that aphonia and aphasia were symptoms of hysteria; he described aphonia in the greatest detail later in the Case of Dora ("Fragment of an Analysis of a Case of Hysteria")[89] and observed aphonia most frequently at the beginning of the nineties when singers with it appeared in his consultation hours.[90]

Of Schnitzler's novella *The Sensitive One* (1895) Beharriell said the "sexual cause of hysteria is presumed to be known." Beharriell continued,

> Undoubtedly Schnitzler has here expressed his conviction, the result of his own immediate experience in the treatment of hysteria, and especially in cases of aphonia. He has even written a special treatise on the hysterical loss of voice, so that one can close in on this disease etiologically and therapeutically.[91]

In the story a doctor advises a singer whose voice has been lost that she should take a lover, and this cures her. The advice does not appear to have originated so much from "that 'uncanny' intuition" which Beharriell ascribed to Schnitzler,[92] or from the work on aphonia, because Schnitzler did not question the etiology of aphonia at all—he did not even suggest it. Schnitzler had another intention:

> The following cases, which must be supplemented in many ways, are notable especially for the therapeutic method of suggestion I have used in them; I do not pretend to present anything essentially new, but to show by several examples the influence of hypnosis and suggestion, a treatment method that still needs further explanation.[93]

This shows how well informed Schnitzler was medically. Freud himself had referred to remarks of Charcot,[94] Chrobak, and Breuer, (whom Schnitzler already knew well at this point) on the sexual etiology of hysteria. Seven years before the appearance of the *Studies on Hysteria* and the novella *The Sensitive One,* Freud wrote in the above-cited lexicon article on hysteria that "functional relationships relating to sexual life play a great role in the etiology of hysteria (as in all other neuroses), and this results from the high psychic meaning of this function."[95] In 1895 Breuer and Freud wrote in their common foreword to the *Studies*:

> Our experiences stem from private practice with an educated, literate[96] social class, and their content touches in many ways the most intimate life and fate of our patients. It would be a gross misuse of trust to publish such communications if there were a danger that the patients would be recognized and facts spread in their circle which were confided to the doctor. We are referring particularly to cases in which sexual and marital circumstances

> have etiological meaning. Therefore we have had to exclude most instructive and convincing observations. From this results the fact that we can bring only very incomplete proof for our view that sexuality plays a leading role in the pathogenesis of hysteria as a source of psychic traumas and a motive for the "defense" for the repression of ideas from consciousness. We even had to exclude the strongly sexual observations from publication.[97]

But in 1893 Breuer and Freud unobtrusively reminded people in their *Preliminary Report* of what they had already observed for years in their patients, namely, how often "painful things" were found "under hypnosis as the basis of hysterial phenomena (the hysterical deleriums of the saints and nuns, of temperate women, of well-brought-up children[98])" and

> that a difficult trauma (as that of a traumatic neurosis), a strenuous suppression (such as of sexual affect), can also bring about a splitting of ideas from affect in an otherwise free person, and this is the mechanism of psychically acquired hysteria.[99]

Something decisive has been said here. The sexual etiology of hysterical symptoms was conjectured, intimated, and rejected among doctors[100] years before Schnitzler's novella *The Sensitive One*. It did not suddenly shoot out of the ground.[101] In a little known letter Breuer wrote:

> Earlier all hysteria was sexual; then we thought we were insulting our patients when we inserted some sort of sexual interpretation into their etiology, and now after the real facts have come out, the pendulum swings to the other side.[102]

One thing is clear: aphonic symptoms were long known to be hysterical manifestations, and the cause was presumed to be in the suppression of the sexual life—thus the connection. But what was not even known in professional circles was the *mechanisms* that governed between sexual life ("painful ideas") and physical symptoms; the *dynamic* that governed between drives and repression (ego defense). What was new[103] for phychoanalysis was the transition from observation and identification of those phenomena to the explanation and understanding[104] of their intrapsychic and psychosomatic functioning.[105] This was shown, for example, in the case history of the singer Rosalia H., a twenty-three year old who complained of aphonic symptoms,[106] in the *Studies*. It was not difficult for Freud to observe here the mechanism of hysterical conversion which he discovered, according to which repressed traumatically affective experiences, principally of the sexual life, caused the physical symptom. Once again the symptom was determined by the traumatic event.

The next step circumscribed the question "which was not possible before psychoanalysis,[107] for earlier one knew nothing of psychic conflict[108] or repression" or how much "the failure of repression" would be "the precondition of symptom formation." But where does such a "repression-demanding opposition between the ego and such individual groups of ideas" come from? Freud asked this question in his short study explaining the problem, *Psychogenic Disturbance of Vision Interpreted Psychoanalytically*[109] where he stated that a primary opposition manifested itself in the conflict of the sexual and ego drives,[110] the latter serving the self-preservation of the individual, the former consisting of partial drives. Freud continued:

> Psychological illumination of our cultural development has taught us that culture exists essentially at the expense of the partial sexual drives, so that these must be suppressed, limited, reformed, and directed to higher goals in order to produce the cultural mental constructs. We could recognize as one valuable result of these investigations what our colleagues still do not want to believe, that the illnesses of men labeled "neuroses" are to be traced back to the manifold means of failure of these reforming processes affecting the partial sexual drives.[111]

Here lies a first answer, whose threads run into the preanalytical time, up to those ideas cited above from the letter to Martha and from the review of Forel's book on hypnotism, in which the connection between drive suppression and cultural development was suggested.

But how might the explanation of the disturbed visual ability be described? Freud wrote:

> The application to the eye and seeing follows easily. When the partial sexual drive which makes use of vision (sexual voyeurism) has drawn to itself the resistance of the ego drives because of its

> excessive claims, so that the ideas by which it strives to express itself become a slave to repression and are kept from consciousness, the relationship of the eye and seeing to the ego and consciousness has been disturbed. The ego has lost its dominance over the organ, which now places itself completely at the service of the repressed drive. . . . It is the revenge, the compensation, of the repressed drive that it, kept from further psychic development, can now increase its dominance over the organ serving it[112]

and causes that symptom of visual disturbance. This connection becomes more obvious whenever "motor organs" (such as hands, fingers, or legs) cease their normal functions under the influence of a repressed drive, possibly for sexual activity, and then show hysterical symptoms of paralysis.

Such a background can also be supposed for the aphonic symptom, particularly because as the moment of "somatic cooperation"[113] that "constitutional part of the disposition to illness" provokes the visual disturbance precisely in that organ.

Because of its time of writing (five years before the turn of the century) as well as its theme, Schnitzler's novella *The Sentimental One* could be considered the transition from the hysterical phenomenon to the drive dynamic. At this time Freud, in the middle of his research, finally parted from the interests of his youth and began *The Interpretation of Dreams,* while Schnitzler turned his back once and for all on his medical routine, for the poet finally silently announced to himself, though without ever giving up contact with his medical colleagues in Vienna and elsewhere, as was fortunate for the cross-fertilization of medicine and the arts. He abandoned his medical profession more openly, but was sought out—more often as he grew older—and asked for advice, as Olga Schnitzler confirmed.[114] For example, his diary noted under May 4, 1921, that Theodor Reik sent a writer patient from his analysis to Schnitzler in order to seek beneficial conversation.

Even after the turn of the century Schnitzler intensively pursued the psychoanalytic developments of Freud and his disciples. He gained an intimate knowledge of psychoanalytic theory[115] through frequent conversations with analysts who knew Freud.[116]

In addition, Schnitzler's *Flirtation* and *Round Dance*[117] also fall within the time when Freud gave lectures on his research and delineations of hysteria, neurasthenia, anxiety neurosis, and obsessional neurosis[118] to the "Viennese Medical Doctors' Colloquium." He noted that he found

> sexual etiology . . . through intensive observation and the study of numerous cases, in about eighty percent of those cases. But what about the factors commonly taken as causes of nervousness (civilization, life in large cities, excessive pressure in schools, the straining of sense organs, the race for acquisition, uncertain life conditions, great catastrophes, the daily intake of poisons)?[119] One must answer that these factors make, in point of fact, no direct contribution to the etiology of neurasthenia. Sexual traumas are the specific causes; they cannot be lacking if a neurosis is to come about. . . . A sexually normal man affected by the other factors does not break down because of them—he does not get any neurosis—while on the other hand these other factors need not be present if only the sexual trauma has an intensive effect long enough.[120]

Krafft-Ebing had gathered sufficient material in the *Psychopathia Sexualis* to support such a claim. Schnitzler reviewed his supplementary work[121] in 1891 and noted that the significance of these investigations may well lie in the fact "that they indicate how false is the position that the law still takes toward those who are sick in their sexual responses."[122] A year earlier Schnitzler touched on the question of "normal" sexuality in relation to ethical social norms:

> We can never be completely sure about the contradictions in the laws that nature on the one hand and society on the other demand. To feel individually means to try to reconcile these contradictions after a fashion.[123]

Significantly, this remark appeared in Schnitzler's major review of Ribbing's *Sexual Hygiene and Its Ethical Consequences* and shows another interest that absorbed the attention of the twenty-eight year old doctor. Schnitzler acknowledged that Ribbing was a learned man, but one with "atavistic prejudices that emerge in him from time to time," although he has almost complete command of "physiology, pathology, and social history." The prejudices concerned the so-called "obscene" literature of authors such as Zola, Strindberg, Garborg, Maupassant, and Hansson,[124] whose harmful effect Ribbing considered more dangerous than that of Boccaccio, Casanova, and Faubla because the contemporary press "trumpets forth" their "clumsy works" as something "outstanding and worthy of imitation." The author of *Anatol* regretted the sadly lacking understanding of art:

> If one were to read Boccaccio, Casanova, Paul de Kock, and then Zola, Strindberg, Krohg, then one would see how differently the idea of sex is developed in the two groups of authors. While in the first group the lust appears in artistic form and a sweet sense of pleasure rules frivolously and adventurously, the other group comes to us in deadly earnest, even covering over the enticing parts of the works with a heavy shadow. Zola's *Blackjack,* Strindberg's *Married,* and Garborg's *The World of Men* are examples of this new world view. Zola and Strindberg did not, of course, write for "foolish youths" who let themselves be " 'tempted to sin' through erotic scenes. Should they have distorted the artistic whole of their production for the sake of these 'readers'?"[125]

The reviewer Schnitzler gradually turned toward the problems that occupied Freud too at this time. To begin with, Schnitzler wrote:

> Björnson demanded not long ago that the husband must approach his future wife just as purely as she approaches him. He dramatically formulated this and the play in question, *The Glove,* produced a lively conflict of opinion. That the men laugh at this demand expressed in the drama as being exaggerated and almost impossible may lie in an arrogance based on a century-old habit; from this behavior one can hardly draw a justified conclusion. But that the women as well cannot suppress a light cheerfulness over the demand of the proud girl in Björnson's drama—that must make one stop and think. For they surely know why they smile.

Previously one read:

> So the question of abstinence might well have been interpreted with too much rigidity in our civilization. But we do not share the opinion that the author takes of diseases originating through abstinence. That these diseases are relatively rarer than those originating through sexual intercourse may well lie in the fact that the young people who are abstinent at a sexually mature age are significantly more rare than those who indulge in sexual intercourse.

Schnitzler's explanations are strikingly similar in tone to Freud's discussion of Averbeck's book on neurasthenia three years before, in 1887, though Freud was clearly directing his review to the medical professional. Freud understood neurasthenia as a "sick state of the nervous system,"

> which may comfortably be described as the most frequent disease in our society, a state which makes most other disease syndromes in the patients of the better classes more complicated and full of consequences. This [neurasthenia] is still not known at all to many scientifically educated doctors or is seen by them simply as a modern name with content added arbitrarily.[126]

Through research that he conducted during the years of Schnitzler's *Flirtation* and *Round Dance* Freud studied the results of abstinence which belong to the etiology of anxiety neurosis.[127]

A few years before his death Freud summarized his work as a doctor in the following words:

> My scientific work set for itself the goal of explaining unusual, abnormal, pathological symptoms of psychic life; that is, of tracing them back to those forces at work behind them and thereby revealing the dynamic mechanisms. I tried this on myself first.[128]

The accents must be placed elsewhere. Beharriell wrote that Schnitzler anticipated the main elements of Freud's *Interpretation of Dreams* in his early literary work *Spring Night in the Dissection Chamber* (1880)—the dream as wish fulfillment, dream censorship, dream displacement, the residue of the day—and later wrote, "Every hypothesis of the Freudian dream theory is fulfilled here."[129]

This is not surprising, for Freud expressly cited as proof of his theories the dreams of creative writers and wrote in *The Interpretation of Dreams*:

> I accidentally discovered in a novella of the poet W. Jensen several artificial dreams that are formed perfectly correctly and could be interpreted as if they were not fictional, but rather had been dreamed by real persons. The poet confirmed after questioning from me that my theory of dreams was unknown to him. I used this agreement between my research and the work of the poet as proof for the correctness of my dream analysis.[130]

In one further point divergences converge. Beharriell told of Schnitzler:

> He began to write down his dreams while still a student or perhaps earlier, long before Freud took an interest in dreams. Schnitzler's literary remains contain more than four hundred pages of sketches of his own dreams from the early eighties until 1927, with scattered interpretive notes.[131]

In several respects we can be more precise. The catalogue of Schnitzler's literary remains shows dream sketches dated as early as 1875;[132] on the other hand, Freud publicly presented his thoughts on the interpretation of dreams for the first time in 1896,[133] though part were formulated a year before in his *Outline of a Psychology.*[134] There the basic idea of the dream as wish fulfillment is found developed scientifically.[135] At the same time attempts to decipher his own dreams in the *Studies on Hysteria* betray Freud's long-awakened interest, symbolically evident in the fact that his famous dream of Irma's injection[137] reaches back into Freud's recollected material in the "cocaine" phase.[138]

But on the other hand it must be made clear what divides the great dream tradition in literature—even that of creative writers. Freud continually supplemented the bibliography in *The Interpretation of Dreams* from the insights of the Freudian interpretation of dreams. He himself wrote,

> With the hypothesis that all dreams may be interpreted I move into immediate contradiction to the prevailing dream theory, even to all dream theories with the exception of Scherner, for to "interpret a dream" means to give it "sense," to replace it through something that fits in as a weighty, equally valuable member in the chain of our psychic action. As we know, prevailing dream theorists allow the scientific theories of dreams no space as problems of dream interpretation, for the dream is not at all a psychic act for them, but a somatic event.[139]

Otto Rank's "basic formula" for Freudian dream interpretation marks the transition from a study of phenomena and observation to a study of dynamics and explanation:

> The dream regularly depicts on the basis, and with the help, of repressed infantile sexual material, actual wishes which are as a rule still erotic, in concealed and symbolically disguised form as fulfilled.[140]

Schnitzler's dream sketches mark exactly that dividing line, which may be fixed for him around the spring of 1900. Under the diary date of March 26, 1900, he wrote of reading Freud's dream interpretation book.[141] Not only did the reading of Freud's work allow Schnitzler to dream "more precisely"—whereby he saw Freud amazingly often in his dreams when he paid close attention—but after that date he interpreted his own and other dreams as well as dreams in fiction in the Freudian manner, and knew how much attention the dream interpreter had to pay to clarifying associations. This differs as well from his own previous practice.[142]

Hardly anyone other than the literary and medical man Schnitzler could have understood better that process of budding psychoanalysis at that time in Vienna—that

> changeover of Freud from physiology to psychology and the step-by-step discovery of the regularities of the unknown psychic life. Further, the abandoning of manipulative and suggestive techniques in treatment in favor of free association and a therapeutic self-reflection methodically put into practice; finally the gradual increase of Freud's self-observation to systematic self-analysis.[143]

The creative writer knew well to separate his nature as "double" in those themes, which Freud indicated to him was common:

> Your determinism like your skepticism—which the people call pessimism[144]—your obsession with the truths of the unconscious, with the instinctive nature of man, your undermining of the conventional cultural securities, the adherence of your thoughts to the polarity of life and death—all that touches me with an uncanny familiarity.[145]

But the difference of talent caused the difference in work. Here ought not to be ascribed in an obliterated or thoughtless way to poetic intuition what stemmed from the realm of information of the doctor or stands out basically from the characteristics of psychoanalytic discoveries.

Freud's modesty, which was described in the beginning of this paper, is illustrated in a dedication that he gave to a few essays he sent to Schnitzler: "With appropriate timidity."[146] But after a visit by Schnitzler to Freud in the freshness of the Berchtesgaden summer two years earlier—the writer had told Freud a dream and spoken of the meaning of the ponds which played a role in some of his works; the analyst spoke of his work *The Ego and the Id* and of the recovery of Gustav Mahler after a consultation—Schnitzler noted on August 16, 1922, in his diary:

> He attracts me again in his whole being, and I experience a certain pleasure in discussing with him all sorts of shallow points of my own work (and existence)—which I prefer to omit.

Timidity here as well? Perhaps also the distance that was never given up by Schnitzler.

NOTES

1. Sigmund Freud, *Briefe 1873-1939* (*Letters 1873-1939*), Frankfurt am Main, 1968, p. 357; and "Briefe an Arthur Schnitzler" ("Letters to Arthur Schnitzler"), ed. and commentated by Heinrich Schnitzler, *Die Neue Rundschau,* Vol. 66, 1955, p. 97.
2. A few years earlier Freud had tried to say something about the psychological explanation of the "double" phenomenon in *Das Unheimliche* (*The Uncanny*) and pointed to Otto Rank's great study on this theme: Cf. Sigmund Freud, *Gesammelte Werke* (*Collected Works*), Imago Edition, Frankfurt am Main, Fischer, Vol. 12, pp. 247f. (Henceforth this edition will be cited as *G.W.*, with the volume and page number.) Gotthart Wunberg has tried to relate this phenomenon to other figures by speaking of "Viennese thought" typical of Freud's and Schnitzler's time. (*Der frühe Hofmannsthal, Schizophrenie als dichterische Struktur* [*The early Hofmannsthal, Schizophrenia as Poetic Structure*], Stuttgart, 1965, pp. 14ff.). Heinz Politzer writes by way of explanation on the "anxiety of the double" on Schnitzler's part: "The writer had become what Freud could have become, if he had not preferred to treat people rather than write about them. The essays which run through the novels of his contemporaries Thomas Mann, Hermann Broch, and Robert Musil are the reverse side of the belles lettres which distinguish Freud's scientific work." ("Freud als Deuter seiner Träume" ["Freud as Interpreter of His Dreams"], *Merkur,* Vol. 24, p. 38.) Interesting in this connection is Schnitzler's diary entry dated about a half year later than Freud's letter, October 22, 1922: "Dr. Asch from New York, Freud disciple,—spoke of the 'elective affinity' between Freud and myself." This entry as well as other quotations cited in this essay from Schnitzler's unpublished diaries are passed on with the kind permission of Heinrich Schnitzler of Vienna.
3. On identification in the work and biography of Freud, see Walter Schönau, *Sigmund Freud's Prosa. Literarische Elemente seines Stils* (*Sigmund Freud's*

Prose: Literary Elements of His Style), Stuttgart, 1968, pp. 115ff. John E. Gedo and Ernest Wolf have pointed to Freud's early characteristic capacity "to identify himself with significant people and to learn from them" on the occasion of the publication of his adolescent correspondence ("Die Ichthyosaurusbriefe" ["The Ichthyosaurus Letters"], *Psyche,* Vol. 24, 1970, pp. 785ff.).

4. Ernest Jones, *Das Leben und Werk von Sigmund Freud* (*The Life and Work of Sigmund Freud*), Vol. 1, Bern, 1960, p. 402.
5. Regarding Freud's relationship to literature, see *Uber Schwierigkeiten im Umgang mit Psychoanalyse und Literatur* (*On Difficulties in Dealing with Psychoanalysis and Literature*), in *Psychoanalyse und Literaturwissenschaft. Texte zur Geschichte ihrer Beziehungen* (*Psychoanalysis and Literary Study: Texts on the History of Their Relationships*), ed. and with intro. by Bernd Urban, Tübingen, 1973, Reihe Deutsche Texte, Vol. 24, pp. xxiiiff.
6. Freud had already written in *Der Dichter und das Phantasieren* (*Creative Writers and Day-Dreaming*), *G.W.,* Vol. 9, p. 150, in 1908: "I have been struck in many of the so-called psychological novels that only one person, namely the hero, is depicted from within. The novelist sits, as it were, in his psyche and looks at the other persons from without. The psychological novel owes its peculiarity to the tendency of the modern novelist to split his ego into partial egos through self-observation, and thus to personify the streams of conflict in his psychic life into several heroes." Robert O. Weiss notes that "far from subscribing uncritically to Freudian ideas in toto, Schnitzler agreed only with those which he found confirmed by his endopsychic perception, his analytical thinking, and his experience." ("The Psychoses in the Works of Arthur Schnitzler," *The German Quarterly,* Vol. 41, 1968, p. 378.) Freud's admiration was aimed at those creative writers "gifted with the ability to pull the most profound insights effortlessly out of the confusion of their own feelings, insights which we have to force our way to only through agonizing insecurity and restless groping." A further passage in Freud touches on another nuance of intuition: "Scientific work is the only way for us which can lead to a knowledge of reality beyond ourselves. It is only an illusion when one expects something from intuition and self-immersion; it can give us nothing beyond explanations—which are hard to interpret—of our own psychic life, never information on those question, the answer to which is so easy for religious teaching." (*G.W.,* Vol. 14, p. 493 [Civilization and Its Discontents]; p. 354 [The Future of an Illusion].
7. *G.W.,* Vol. 7, p. 69 (Delusion and Dream in Jensen's *Gradiva*).
8. See Frederick J. Beharriell, "Schnitzler's Anticipation of Freud's Dream Theory," *Monatshefte für Deutschunterricht,* Vol. 45, 1953, pp. 81ff.; "Schnitzler: Freud's Doppelgänger" ("Schnitzler: Freud's Double"), *Literatur und Kritik,* Vol. 2, 1967, pp. 546ff. (Following quote: pp. 547ff.) Richard H. Allen had noted previously in his bibliography to Robert O. Weiss's dissertation *A Study of Arthur Schnitzler*: "Arthur Schnitzler was far ahead of his time in depth psychology" (*An Annotated Arthur Schnitzler Bibliography,* Chapel Hill, N.C., 1966, p. 127).
9. Actually the *Studies on Hysteria* by Breuer and Freud first appeared six years later. Hartmut Scheible is also of the opinion that "Schnitzler in his treatise 'Ueber funktionelle Aphonie und deren Behandlung durch Hypnose und Suggestion' ('On Functional Aphonia and Its Treatment by Hypnosis and Suggestion'), 1889, preceded Breuer's and Freud's hysteria studies by four years" (*Diskretion und Verdrängung. Zu Schnitzlers Autobiographie.* [*Discretion and Repression. On Schnitzler's Autobiography*], *Frankfurter Hefte,* Vol. 25, 1970, p. 130). Recently, Heinze Rieder noted that Schnitzler "had printed a scientific work which was important to his intellectual

development" in his work on aphonia (*Arthur Schnitzler. Das dramatische Werk* [*Arthur Schnitzler: The Dramatic Work*], Vienna, 1973, p. 18). See also Theodor W. Alexander, "The Author's Debt to the Physician: Aphonia in the Works of Arthur Schnitzler, *Journal of the Arthur Schnitzler Research Association*, Vol. 4, No. 4, 1964, pp. 4ff.

10. R. Müller-Freienfels speaks of the fact that "an exact treatment of the relationship between Freud and Schnitzler" is still lacking (in his Frankfurt dissertation of 1954, *Das Lebensgefühl in Arthur Schnitzlers Dramen* [*The Feeling of Life in Arthur Schnitzler's Dramas*]). "Especially the question of when the writer was influenced by Freud and how much he himself anticipated him has remained unclarified." Oskar Walzel writes in his *Handbuch der Literaturwissenschaft* (*Handbook of Literary Studies*): "Schnitzler's conscious relationship to Freud and psychoanalysis is that much closer. At the time when he was still a practicing scientific doctor, Schnitzler went Breuer's way and wanted to treat functional aphonia with hypnosis and suggestion. As a creative writer he came closer and closer to Freud's notions of psychic disturbances. Freud himself granted Schnitzler's *Paracelsus* deep insights into the psychic mechanism of the motives of illness" (see note 5, p. 128). One can read on this drama, which originated two years after the publication of the Freud-Breuer hysteria studies, in the *Deutsch-Oesterreichischen Literaturgeschichte* (*German-Austrian Literary History*) by Nagl-Zeidler-Castle (Vol. 4, p. 1756): "Under Freud's direct influence, Schnitzler at once gained a close feeling for the real concerns of psychoanalysis. Even the first verse-play presented how psychic agitation, which may not pass the threshhold of the censor whose presence the waking consciousness can and will not admit to itself, becomes extremely clear in dreams: Paracelsus then anticipates the theory of rendering harmless (abreaction) the memories (repressed complexes) which have become pathogenic." Practically at the same time, Richard Plaut alleges in his Basel dissertation (*Arthur Schnitzler als Erzähler* [*Arthur Schnitzler as Story-teller*], 1935, p. 16) that Schnitzler continually refused to "consciously use the results of psychoanalysis in his works, to place on them an artistic garment which concealed only incompletely the theorems of his method. If one does not take into account the extremely orthodox interpretations of psychoanalysis, psychic cases result which resemble those of Freud only marginally. On the problem of the "anticipation" of psychoanalytic insights and ideas, see note 5, pp. xviiff. Gerd Klaus Schneider attempts to maintain in his dissertation that Nietzsche's philosophy provided backgorund for influences common to both Schnitzler and Freud. Factually and chronologically, this is hardly conclusive for the period which we are investigating and hardly goes beyond analogies. (*Arthur Schnitzler und die Psychologie seiner Zeit, unter besonderer Berücksichtigung der Philosophie Friedrich Nietzsches* (*Arthur Schnitzler and the Psychology of His Time, Especially Considered with Friedrich Nietzsche's Philosophy*), dissertation, Washington, D.C., 1968).

11. *G.W.*, Vol. 13, pp. 357f [Josef Popper-Lynkeus and the Theory of Dreams],

12. See note 4, pp. 402f.

13. Another director of the Burg Theater, Burkhard, had written a rather negative review of *The Interpretation of Dreams* shortly before its appearance. See *Psyche*, Vol. 26, 1972, p. 708.

14. See *Almanach der Psychoanalyse*, 1933, p. 288. On the references to the thoughts on the Aristotelian theory of catharsis which are developed in the *Studies on Hysteria* and on Hermann Bahr's *Dialog vom Tragischen* (*Dialogue of the Tragic*), see note 5, p. 58.

15. On the "various levels of consciousness" see Schnitzler's statements in

Psychologische Literatur: "One discovered, furthermore, and this was perhaps the most essential thing, a kind of fluctuating no-man's land between consciousness and the subconscious. The subconscious does not begin as immediately as one believes, or sometimes pretends to believe out of convenience (an error which the psychoanalyst cannot always avoid). The art of the creative writer will consist of drawing the boundary between the conscious, the half-conscious, and the unconscious as sharply as possible." (*Gesammelte Werke. Aphorismen und Betrachtungen* [*Aphorisms and Observations*], ed. by Robert O. Weiss, Frankfurt am Main, 1967, p. 455). Heinz Politzer, for example, sees this "art of the creative writer" at work in Schnitzler's *Leutnant Gustl.* [*Diagnose und Dichtung. Zum Werk Arthur Schnitzlers,* in *Das Schweigen der Sirenen* (*Diagnosis and Poetry: On Arthur Schnitzler's Works,* in *Silence of the Sirens*), Stuttgart, 1968, p. 121]. But Breuer's statements are aimed precisely at that "fluctuating no-man's land" in the *Studies on Hysteria,* e.g., in the chapters "Hypnoid States" and "Unconscious Ideas and Ideas Inadmissible to Consciousness—Splitting of the Psyche" (S. Freud and J. Breuer, *Studien über Hysterie,* Frankfurt am Main, Fischer Taschenbuch, 1970, Vol. 6001, pp. 173f. Only this newer edition also contains Breuer's contributions, but for some strange reason forgoes a printing of the significant foreword to the 1895 edition.) Freud sketches out these lines in his description of the "psychic apparatus," a system in which the unconscious has access to consciousness only through the preconscious. This theory is already found in *The Interpretation of Dreams,* which appeared in Winter 1899 (*G.W.,* Vols. 2-3, pp. 542ff.) but may be traced back years before that and experience later additions, expansion, and changes (see the notes to the study edition of the *Traumdeutung,* Frankfurt am Main, 1972, Vol. 2, pp. 517ff.). Likewise around 1898 Freud writes *Ueber Deckerinnerungen* (*Screen Memories*) and reports of a childhood memory—children picking flowers—which strongly resembled a scene remembered in Schnitzler (see Herbert I. Kupper and Hilda S. Rollman-Branch, "Freud und Schnitzler—Doppelgänger," *Journal of the American Psychoanalytic Association,* Vol. 7, 1959, p. 120). Freud writes in the introduction to *Deckerinnerungen* (*G.W.,* Vol. 1, p. 531) how often he had to bother with "fragments of memories . . . which had remained for the individual in his memory from the first years of childhood, and one had to claim a large pathogenic meaning for the impressions of this time of life." These insights go—via *The Interpretation of Dreams*—to the theory of infantile sexuality, about which Schnitzler exhibited strong scepticism. Politzer points to this in the above passage (p. 130), although, on the other hand, an infantile trauma has an indirect effect in the story *Der Sohn* (*The Son,* 1892). (See Robert O. Weiss, "The Psychoses in the Works of Arthur Schnitzler," *The German Quarterly,* Vol. 41, 1968, p. 392.) With the other characteristic of later psychoanalysis cited by Beharriell, "the dominance of the unconscious over the conscious," it has already been considered by Freud how the unconscious on the one hand stands in a philosophical (and literary) tradition, but on the other differs essentially from that which the attributes to him. See note 5, pp. xixff.

16. Sigmund Freud, *G.W.,* Vol. 7 [Delusion and Dream in Jensen's *Gradiva*], p. 70. Likewise the following quote.
17. Freud knew virtually the complete works of this author. See also "Meine Berührung mit Josef Popper-Lynkeus" ("My Contact with Josef Popper-Lynkeus"), *G.W.,* Vol. 16, pp. 261ff., and *Briefe 1873-1939,* Frankfurt am Main, 1968, pp. 329f.
18. See note 11.

19. See "Psychoanalyse als Archäologie der Seele" ("Psychoanalysis as an Archaeology of the Psyche") in Walter Schönau, *op. cit.* Jack J. Spector reports recently on Freud's love for archaeology and on his art objects in the London house: *Freud und die Aesthetik. Psychoanalyse, Literatur, und Kunst* (*Freud and Aesthetics: Psychoanalysis, Literature, and Art*), Munich, 1973, pp. 21ff.
20. See esp. Freud's adolescent correspondence (in *Psyche.,* Vol. 24, 1970, pp. 768ff.) and Heinz Stanescu, "Ein Gelegenheitsgedicht des jungen Freud" ("An Occasional Poem of the Young Freud"), in *Deutsch für Ausländer. Informationen für die Lehrer,* 1967, pp. 13ff., and "Unbekannte Briefe des jungen Sigmund Freud an einen rumänischen Freund" ("Unknown Letters of the Young Freud to a Roumanian Friend") in *Neue Literatur. Zeitschrift des Schriftstellerverbandes der Sozialistischen Republik Rumänien,* Vol. 16, 1965, pp. 123ff.
21. See Sigmund Freud, *Selbstdarstellung. Schriftenz ur Geschichte der Psychoanalyze* (*Self-portrait: Writings on the History of Psycho-Analysis*), ed. and with intro. by I. Grubrich-Simitis, Frankfurt am Main, Fischer Taschenbuch, 1971, Vol. 6096, p. 106. Likewise the following quote.
22. Arthur Schnitzler, *Jugend in Wien. Eine Autobiographie* (*Youth in Vienna: An Autobiography*), Ed. by Th. Nickl and H. Schnitzler, Munich, 1971, dtv-Taschenbuch, Vol. 775, p. 27.
23. Heinz Rieder points to the allusions to literature in this unusual technical work (*op. cit.,* p. 15), which Schnitzler received as a gift from his father "as was proper right after his successful final exams, with a tender dedication." It remained, however, "at first unread" (see note 22, p. 82).
24. The diary notes under January 17, 1890: "My aversion to the public, to doctors, practice, medicine, has risen considerably; thinking of the future, I shudder. My literary ambitions not well received at home . . . still no successes to show. Too bad (they say); that a doctor, a practicing doctor, writes poems, one may not know. . . . My course is clear to me, though. Inwardly, I am through with medicine. I know, rather late, that I am no good at all for it. I am disgusted by patients and my colleagues, above all by what reminds me of the profession."
25. See Schnitzler's reviews of Meynert's "Klinische Volesungen über Psychiatrie" ("Clinical Lectures on Psychiatry") in *Internationale Klinische Rundschau,* Vol. 5, 1891, col. 162. Meynert was also Freud's teacher. Schnitzler's diary notation of June 16, 1922, states how the writer conversed with Freud on "hospital and military times" and "common bosses": common teachers were the anatomist Langer, the physiologist Brücke, the chemist Ludwig, the zoologist Claus, and possibly Breuer, who in 1877-78 lectured on kidney diseases. See note 22, p. 83, and Siegfried Bernfeld, "Sigmund Freud M.D. 1882-85," *International Journal of Psycho-Analysis,* Vol. 32, 1951, pp. 216f. On the medical schools in Vienna at that time, see M. Dorer, *Historische Grundlagen der Psychoanalyse* (*Historical Bases of Psychoanalysis*), Leipzig, 1932, pp. 112ff.
26. See note 22, p. 236. In the *Fragmentary Novel,* whose beginnings go back to a sketch on the novel *Wurstel: A Viennese Novel* of 1896, it is said of Dr. Rudolf Forlan, assistant doctor in the general hospital, that "he dutifully followed the professor during visits, reported on the patients personally assigned to him, attended the lecture and thus also the presentation of one of the patients, and made the listeners familiar with the case history. He saw in the cool glance which the professor occasionally cast over him once again the complete indifference to his person. That the great scholar didn't think much of him was known to him and even to his assistant, Dr. Lüdemann. Rudolf was hardly a colleague to be taken seri-

ously, but rather a young man from a good family who, as the son of a doctor, without a real inner calling, had likewise studied medicine and had been accidentally assigned to the psychiatric ward, as he had been assigned to the internal ward in the six months previous." (*Literatur und Kritik,* Vol. 2, 1967, p. 151).

27. The eighty-year-old Freud impressively relates why he and his brother did not allow themselves a trip to Greece: "It was connected with the constriction and poverty of the circumstances of our lives. It has to be that a guilt feeling was tied to the satisfaction of having brought it so far. There is something in that, something wrong which has been forbidden from ancient times. It has something to do with the child's criticism of his father, with the disdain which the overestimation of his person in early childhood had set loose. It looks as if the essential thing in success is to go further than the father, as if it were still not permitted to want to surpass him. To this generally applicable motivation may be added for our case the special circumstance, that there is a reference to the superiority of the sons contained in the theme of Athens and the Acropolis. Our father was a businessman who had not completed high school. Athens could not mean much to him. What disturbed us about enjoying a trip to Athens was thus a stirring of filial piety." (*G.W.,* Vol. 16 [A Disturbance of Memory on the Acropolis], pp. 256f.)
28. See note 22, p. 240.
29. See note 22, p. 247.
30. See note 26. Dr. Forlan likewise lectures "not without scientific interest in Charcot" (*op. cit.,* p. 139).
31. See note 22, p. 284. Cf. Theodor W. Alexander, "The Author's Debt to the Physician: Aphonia in the Works of Arthur Schnitzler," *Journal of the International Arthur Schnitzler Research Association,* Vol. 4, 1965, No. 4, pp. 4ff.
32. Dr. Forlan likewise performs hypnotic experiments (see note 26, p. 171). Felix Salten was also a witness of Schnitzler's hypnotic experiments. He reports about them extensively in his memoirs "From the Beginnings" (*Jahrbuch deutscher Bibliophilen und Literaturfreunde,* Vols. 18-19, 1932-33, pp. 33f.)
33. See note 26. Dr. Forlan felt that his "hypnotic experiments were only a game" and had to be advised by his father, who likewise was a doctor, to "occupy himself rather with the exact areas of his science," and, in particular, "to turn again to his histological work" (*op. cit.,* p. 165). One is struck by the similarity of Ernst Brücke's advice to Freud, who had remained "stuck in physiology," that he should avoid a theoretical career. Freud writes: "Thus I came from the histology of the nervous system to neuropathology and eventually to a concern with neuroses." (*G.W.,* Vol. 14 [Postscript to Discussion on Lay Analysis], pp. 290f.)
34. Thus Schnitzler attached great importance to correcting the mistake of having been named co-worker of the great *Klinischer Atlas der Laryngologie und Rhinologie* (*Clinical Atlas of Laryngology and Rhinology*), which his father had edited since 1891 with Hajek, "as he had contributed practically nothing to the atlas" (Richard H. Allen, *op. cit.,* p. 84).
35. On the doctor figures in the narrative works, see Hans Wiedenbrüg, *Die literarischen Motive in der erzählenden Kunst Arthur Schnitzlers* (*Literary Motives in Schnitzler's Narrative Works*), Frankfurt am Main, 1934, and Reinhart Müller-Freienfels, *Das Lebensgefühl in Arthur Schnitzlers Dramen* (*The Attitude Toward Life in Arthur Schnitzler's Dramas*), dissertation, Frankfurt am Main, 1954, p. 3. Schnitzler's statement, "I was born in 1862 and was a physician," is cited here as well. Olga Schnitzler relates the fol-

lowing opinion by Schnitzler of himself: "I will not be remembered so much as a creative writer, much more rather as a strange subject of cultural history." (*Spiegelbild der Freundschaft* [*Mirror-Image of Friendship*], Salzburg, 1962, p. 137.) One might see in these statements, which can be compounded by diary notations, a faltering of creative self-confidence, which sought again and again to adhere to and orient itself to the medical profession. Gerd Klaus Schneider quotes in this connection from Schnitzler's letter of July 11, 1927, to Josef Körner, in which the writer says that he "counts himself according to intellectual disposition not to creative writers but rather to the natural scientists (writers with a predominantly psychological attitude)" (*op. cit.*, pp. 311f.). Françoise Derré's chapter "Schnitzler, Man of Science" (*L'oeuvre d'Arthur Schnitzler*, Paris, 1966, pp. 196ff.) is summarized in Freud's incisive remark, "Schnitzler is not only a creative writer but also a scientist" (G. S. Viereck, "An Interview with Freud," *Psychoanalysis*, Vol. 4, 1955-57, p. 10). From this medical-professional confidence stems Schnitzler's critique of Werfel's "Schweiger" ("Taciturn"), which begins with the words: "A rather bizarre case history, in no way corresponding to medical experience of psychopathology, carried out arbitrarily in both a medical and a poetic sense," (*Gesammelte Werke. Aphorismen und Betrachtungen*, Frankfurt am Main, 1967, p. 491). Characteristic for the poet, who was constantly orienting himself medically and maintaining numerous medical contacts, is the following diary passage of September 27, 1922: "Cottage sanatorium. Diathermia. Dr. Liebesny shows me apparatus. Dr. Wittels as well. Medical conversations on the effect of psychic events on physical—origin of "willful" organic diseases (in which I do not believe)."

36. In 1927 Freud wrote in retrospect: "In my youth, the need to understand something of the riddles of the world and perhaps even to contribute something to their solution became overpowering. Enrollment on the medical faculty seemed the best way." (*G.W.*, Vol. 14 [Postscript to Discussion on Lay Analysis], p. 290.)
37. See note 1, p. 57.
38. See also Friedrich Heer, "Explosionen. Wien und sein Untergrund" ("Explosions: Vienna and Its Underground"), *Emuna*, Vol. 8, 1973, pp. 83ff.
39. Hartmut Scheible remarks in his thoughts on Schnitzler's autobiography, *Jugend in Wien* (*Youth in Vienna*): "He conceals as much as he reveals in his autobiography. . . . Not that a characteristic of an especially pronounced ego or character weakness can be found in Schnitzler; rather, there is the sense that Schnitzler leaves his 'innermost ego' so consistently in the dark that his memoirs seem strangely impersonal despite all the richness of material and intimate detailing. . . . As openly as Schnitzler relates, he nonetheless avoids with discretion worthy of a Grillparzer, extending the dangers which he sees himself struck by or flirts with them wordily." ("Diskretion und Verdrängung. Zu Schnitzlers Autobiographie" ["Discretion and Repression: On Schnitzler's Autobiography], *Frankfurter Hefte*, Vol. 25, 1970, p. 133f.)
40. *G.W.*, Vols. 2-3 (*The Interpretation of Dreams*), p. x.
41. See note 21, p. 24.
42. *G.W.*, Vol. 2-3 (The Interpretation of Dreams), p. viii.
43. See in this connection Heinz Politzer, "Freud als Deuter seiner Träume" ("Freud as Interpreter of His Dreams"), *Merkur*, Vol. 24, 1970, pp. 34ff., and Jack Spector, note 19, pp. 110ff. H. Kupper and H. Rollmann-Branch (see note 15, p. 116) connect *The Interpretation of Dreams* in Freud's biography to Schnitzler's novel *Der Weg ins Freie* (*Into the Open*). Schnitzler spoke of the latter as one of his "most personal creations" (see *Hugo*

von Hofmannsthal—Arthur Schnitzler: Briefwechsel [*Correspondence*], Frankfurt am Main, 1964, p. 257).

44. See the works of Reik, Sachs, and Storfer named by Allen (note 8).
45. See note 21, pp. 9ff.
46. *G.W.*, Vol. 2-3 (The Interpretation of Dreams), p. viii.
47. See note 20 and S. Freud, *Braubriefe* (*Bridal Letters*), Frankfurt am Main, Fischer Taschenbuch, 1968, Vol. 899.
48. See note 21, p. 9.
49. Almost at the same time that Schnitzler begins his diary, which encompasses thousands of pages, Freud comes to his "primal analysis" with his "alter ego" in his friend Fliess. See M. Mannoni, *Der Psychiater, sein Patient und die Psychoanalyse* (*The Psychiatrist, His Patients, and Psycho-Analysis*), Frankfurt am Main, 1973, pp. 198f.
50. Franz Werfel, "Arthur Schnitzler," *Die Neue Rundschau,* Vol. 43, 1932, p. 3.
51. See the survey of these works in Allen, note 8, pp. 83ff., and Gerhard Neumann and Jutta Müller, *Der Nachlass Arthur Schnitzlers* (*Arthur Schnitzler's Literary Remains*), Munich, 1969, pp. 119ff. and 155.
52. *Wiener Medizinische Presse,* Vol. 27, 1886, col. 1665 (not named by Allen, Note 8).
53. Vol. 1, 1887, cols. 19f.
54. *Wiener Medizinische Wochenschrift,* 1886, cols. 1445ff.
55. *Ibid.,* cols. 1633ff.
56. See note 53.
57. See *G.W.*, Vol. 14 (*An Autobiographical Study*), pp. 39f.
58. See note 21, p. 47 (n. 23).
59. See note 52.
60. See note 53.
61. *Internationale Klinische Rundschau,* Vol. 3, 1889, col. 893.
62. *Ibid.*, Vol. 6, 1892, cols. 2133 and 1887.
63. *Ibid.*, Vol. 3, 1889, cols. 407 and 584.
64. *Ibid.*, Vol. 1, 1887, cols. 185ff., and *Wiener Medizinische Wochenschrift,* 1887, col. 138.
65. See also Jürgen vom Scheidt, "Sigmund Freud und das Kokain" ("Sigmund Freud and Cocaine"), *Psyche,* Vol. 27, 1973, pp. 385ff.
66. Erlenmeyer names, after reports of cases of cocaine poisoning increased everywhere in the world, this drug, next to alcohol and morphine, as the "third scourge of mankind" (see note 65, p. 393).
67. *Internationale Klinische Rundschau,* Vol. 2, 1883, cols. 22f. (not named by Allen, Note 8).
68. Jürgen vom Scheidt demonstrates in his large study what meaning Freud's concern with addiction and cocaine had for the origin and development of psychoanalysis. In this connection also see Freud's later statements in his critical writings on culture, which show how recreation, substitute gratifications, narcotics, art, and religion are aids in making the severity of life bearable. In 1897 Freud writes to Fliess: "The insight has occurred to me that masturbation is the sole great habit, the 'original addiction," the substitution and release of which brings about the other addictions (to alcohol, morphine, tobacco, etc.). The role of this addiction is immense in hysteria" (see note 65, p. 409).
69. See note 67.
70. Like Dr. Rudolf Forlan (see note 32), Paracelsus and later Fridolin in *Traumnovelle* (*Dream Novel*) practice hypnotism. All of them, as well as Anatol, want to call up the past into the present or find truth behind ap-

pearance, and that over and beyond the control of memory, which plays an extraordinary role both in the *Studies on Hysteria* and in many works of Schnitzler. See Müller-Freienfels, *op. cit.*, pp. 51ff., and Heinz Rieder, *op. cit.*, p. 31.

71. See *Gesammelte Werke. Die dramatischen Werke,* Vol. 1, Frankfurt am Main, 1962, pp. 34ff.
72. Freud describes here already the opposition which is later to be directed against basic concepts of psychoanalysis, e.g., "against the hypothesis of a dynamically effective unconscious psychic life, i.e., a theory which puts an end to the fiction of the 'free will' of man, and amounts to the assertion 'that the ego is no longer master in its own house' " (Anna Freud, *Schwierigkeiten der Psychoanalyse in Vergangenheit und Gegenwart [Difficulties of Psychoanalysis in the Past and Present]*, Frankfurt am Main, 1972, p. 12). On the problem of determinism, of free will, and of causality in Schnitzler, which also gives background for Freud, see Müller-Freienfels, *op. cit.*, pp. 66ff., and Gerd Klaus Schneider, *op. cit.*, pp. 315ff. See also note 76.
73. *Wiener Medizinische Wochenschrift,* 1889, col. 1099, also Standard Edition, Vol. 1.
74. *G.W.*, Vol. 1 (*Studies on Hysteria*), p. 265.
75. See note 5, p. xli, and Maud Mannoni, note 49, p. 201.
76. See note 72. In addition, it is significant that Hermann Bahr writes in 1891 in his essay "Die neue Psychologie" ("The New Psychology") that this must be "deterministic. . . . Thus there are no loose people floating freely in the air, one doesn't know from where, why and where to, as in the old psychologies; rather, they are chained to their development and surroundings, which is their fate. We leave the naturalistic models, but we can never leave the milieu. We will always place every individual feeling in relationship to all feelings, even in relationship to its origins and conditions, which condition it. We proceed thus just as naturalism had to, when it proceeded at all psychologically" (*Zur Uberwindung des Naturalismus. Theoretische Schriften 1887 bis 1904 [On Overcoming Naturalism: Theoretical Writings, 1887-1904]*, sel., intro., and annot. by Gotthart Wunberg, Stuttgart, 1968, p. 56). Freud was already at work when Bahr demanded of the new psychology in the same passage that it must be "decompositive . . . in that the additions, postscripts, and all reworkings of the consciousness are separate, and feelings are traced back to their original appearance in consciousness. The old psychology finds only the least effective feelings, whose expression is formulated in the end by consciousness and retained by memory. The new psycholology of will seeks its primary elements, its beginnings in the obscurities of the soul, before they surface through this very time-consuming, involved, and confusedly intricate process of feeling, which throws complicated facts over the threshold of consciousness, in the end becoming simple conclusions."
77. Volhard has already pointed out references in literary productions to "free association" (see note 5, pp. 111f.); for those in *Leutnant Gustl* see H. Kupper and H. Rollman-Branch, note 15, p. 114.
78. See note 21, pp. 8ff.; note 4, pp. 288ff., and *G.W.*, Vol 1 (*Studies on Hysteria*), pp. 201ff.
79. See note 63, col. 586.
80. See *G.W.*, Vol. 1 (*Studies on Hysteria*), pp. 296ff.
81. See *G.W.*, Vol. 13 ("A Short Account of Psychoanalysis"), p. 410.
82. H. H. Meyer reports on his scientific development, immense education, and friendship with Marie von Ebner-Eschenbach in *Neue Oesterreichische Biographie* (*New Austrian Biography*), Vol. 5, 1928, pp. 30ff. The early phase of the connection with Freud is investigated by Nathan Schlessinger,

"The Scientific Style of Breuer and Freud in the Origins of Psychoanalysis," *Journal of the American Psychoanalytic Association,* Vol. 15, 1967, pp. 404ff.

83. See also Frederick M. Bram, "Das Geschenk der Anna O." ("The Gift of Anna O."), *Psyche,* Vol. 27, 1973, pp. 449ff.
84. *G.W.,* Vol. 13 ("A Short Account of Psychoanalysis"), p. 408.
85. *Studien über Hysterie* (see Note 15), pp. 176f. Connections can be made from this point to the sick Marie, who is bound to her father in the opening scene of *Der Ruf des Lebens* (*Call of Life*). Hertha Krotkoff relates Marie's fate to that of Marianne in the *Traumnovelle*: both sacrifice their youth to the care of a sick father, but "the starting point of the drama was taken up in a negative variation in the *Traumnovelle* as an episode with a very specific function." See "Themen, Motive und Symbole in Arthur Schnitzlers *Traumnovelle*" ("Themes, Motives, and Symbols in Arthur Schnitzler's *Dream Novel*), *Modern Austrian Literature,* Vol. 5, 1972, p. 84.
86. See note 85, p. 27.
87. *G.W.,* Vol. 13 ("A Short Account of Psychoanalysis"), pp. 407, 409.
88. See A. Villaret, *Handwörterbuch der gesamten Medizin* (*Hand Dictionary of Total Medicine*), Stuttgart, 1888, p. 888.
89. *G.W.,* Vol. 5 ("Fragment of an Analysis of a Case of Hysteria"), pp. 199f.
90. *G.W.,* Vol. 1 (*Studies on Hysteria*), p. 237. Schnitzler's father was for a time active as a "professor of physiology and pathology of voice and speech at the Vienna conservatory." See Ludwig Eisenberg, *Das geistige Wien* (*Intellectual Vienna*), Vol. 2, Vienna, 1893, p. 424.
91. See note 8, p. 553.
92. See note 91.
93. See note 63, col. 405. This stated intention may somewhat modify Heinz Rieder's opinion that Schnitzler's aphonia essay was a "scientific work which was important for his intellectual development" (*op. cit.,* p. 18).
94. See Léon Chertok, "Freud in Paris (1885/86)," *Psyche,* Vol. 27, 1973, p. 441.
95. See note 88, pp. 889f.
96. This circumstance placed high demands on the degree of education; see notes 3, 5, and 82, and *Marie von Ebner-Eschenbach—Josef Breuer: Ein Briefwechsel. 1889-1916,* ed. by Robert A. Kann, Vienna, 1969.
97. *G.W.,* Vol. 1 (*Studies on Hysteria*), p. 77.
98. In Freud's posthumous writings we read: ". . . of persons who feel tendencies to art and the theater in themselves." See *G.W.,* Vol. 17 ("On the Theory of Hysterical Attacks), p. 12.
99. *G.W.,* Vol. 1 (*Studies on Hysteria*), pp. 89, 92.
100. Charcot, for example, had declared to his colleagues that the origin of hysteria was "that genital thing," but in the official theory he keeps the sexual factor to a minimum. See note 94, p. 447. Breuer and Freud parted ways on this point during the period that followed. Jack Spector writes: "Moreover, a series of psychoanalytical themes, for example, infantile sexuality and the sexual etiology of neurosis, were frequently subjects of discussion in the psychiatric circles in fin de siècle Paris" (*op. cit.,* p. 30).
101. In parallel fashion, Peter Altenberg's letter to Schnitzler of 1895 offers a good example of "anticipation" of psychoanalytic knowledge, of the idea of sublimation, and of the striving for compensation on the part of inferior organs: "Believe me, Dr. Arthur, we poor people are like certain patients. Certain organs refine themselves, increase their efficiency in order to cover up the deficiency of others. So it is with potency in every form. Economic forces, sexual forces are compensated by higher ones. The brain, as it were,

takes over their duties, takes advantage of the atrophy." (Quoted by Schneider, *op. cit.*, pp. 87f.)

102. *Gesnerus,* Vol. 14, 1957, p. 171. A misunderstanding obviously still current may be pointed out. Heinz Rieder remarks that Schnitzler did not follow Freud in a one-sided theory of drive which traces everything back to sexual drives (*op. cit.*, p. 18). Freud defended himself often against this incorrect representation of his theory. He writes, for example: "Psychoanalysis has never forgotten that there are also nonsexual motive forces. It is constructed on the sharp separation of sexual drives from ego drives and asserts before each objection, not that the neuroses arise from sexuality, but rather that they owe their origin to the conflict between ego and sexuality." See *G.W.*, Vol. 11 (*Introductory Lectures on Psycho-Analysis*), p. 364.
103. See also note 76.
104. For these ideas, see note 5, p. xxvi.
105. See S. Freud: "Confirmation of a phenomenon naturally immediately brings up the question of its causality." (*G.W.*, Vol. 16 [A Disturbance of Memory on the Acropolis], p. 252). As far as I know this difference—related to Schnitzler—has only been described by Lotte S. Couch ("*Der Reigen*: Schnitzler und Sigmund Freud," *Oesterreich in Geschichte und Literatur,* Vol. 16, 1972, p. 225): "While Freud is interested in the origin of complex psychic structures and pursues these back to their early beginnings, Schnitzler describes the finished product, the complicated psyche with all its variegated reactions to the circumstances of the present. Let us make this concrete in the example of the married couple. Schnitzler doesn't tell us why the man from 'better circles' sees in sexual intercourse with his own wife an injuring of the sacrament of marriage, and how this notion could originate in him. But Freud follows this behavior of man which presently manifests itself back into its early beginnings and makes an effort to discover its genesis, thus discovering, in this case, the significance of the mother as a longed-for sexual object, likewise forbidden by the barrier of the incest taboo. As Schnitzler does not deal with the genesis of psychic structures of his characters, one brings with psychoanalysis a further dimension to his work, that of temporal depth."
106. See *G.W.*, Vol. 1 (*Studies on Hysteria*), pp. 237ff.
107. Significant in this connection is Freud's statement on Ernst Mach, which is found in a letter to Josef Popper-Lynkeus on August 4, 1916: "Your beautiful, enviable appreciation of your late friend Mach was already known to me as a reader of the *Vossische Zeitung*. I had, unfortunately, not found a way to him from my more narrow point of view and had to find his way of dealing with psychic things unpsychological. The physicist and psychologist come together only with difficulty" (*Briefe 1873-1939,* Note 1, p. 330).
108. On "psychological" and "emotional" conflict and references to literature, see H. Kupper and H. Rollman-Branch, note 15, pp. 117f.
109. *G.W.*, Vol. 8 ("The Psychoanalytic View of Psychogenic of Vision Disturbances"), pp. 94ff.
110. See note 102.
111. See note 109, p. 98.
112. See note 109, p. 99.
113. See note 109, p. 102.
114. Olga Schnitzler, *op. cit.*, p. 138.
115. Otto P. Schinnerer wrote already in 1933 in connection with Schnitzler's *Buch der Sprüche und Bedenken* (*Book of Sayings and Scruples*): "Highly illuminating is a series of notes on psychoanalysis, in which he takes sharp issue with some of the dogmas of the orthodox school" ("Arthur Schnitz-

ler's 'Nachlass,'" *The Germanic Review,* Vol. 8, 1933, p. 119). See also Arthur Schnitzler, *Gesammelte Werke. Aphorismen und Betrachtungen,* pp. 267ff., and "On Psychoanalysis" (*Protokolle, Wiener Halbjahresschrift,* Nr. 2, 1976, pp. 277 ff.) See also Hartmut Schieble, *A. Schnitzler und die Aufklarung* (*A.S. and the Enlightenment*), Munchen, 1977.

116. See also Schnitzler's published diaries, note 2.
117. See also the work of Lotte S. Couch in note 105.
118. Robert O. Weiss apparently overlooks in his essay "The Psychoses in the Work of Arthur Schnitzler" (*The German Quarterly,* Vol. 41, 1968, pp. 377ff.) the fact that Freud undertook at this time the epoch-making division of neurosis and psychosis and already speaks of psychosis in numerous differentiations. See *G.W.,* Vol. 1 ("The Neuro-Psychoses of Defence" and *Studies on Hysteria*), pp. 69, 72f., 123, 262.
119. On the individual arguments see also Willy Hellpach, *Nervosität und Kultur* (*Nervousness and Culture*), Berlin, 1902.
120. S. Freud, "Ueber Hysterie," *Wiener Medizinische Presse,* Vol. 36, 1895, col. 1640.
121. *Neue Forschungen auf dem Gebiete der Psychopathia sexualis: Eine medizinisch-psychologische Studie* (*New Research in the Area of Psychopathia Sexualis: A Medical-Psychological Study*), Stuttgart, 1890.
122. *Internationale Klinische Rundschau,* Vol. 5, 1891, col. 70.
123. *Ibid.,* Vol. 4, 1890, col. 1939.
124. On the significance of these authors, see the theoretical writings of Hermann Bahr cited in note 76.
125. See note 123, col. 1937ff. See also Schnitzler's later statements on "dirty literature" and "pornography" in *Gesammelte Werke. Aphorismen und Betrachtungen,* pp. 324f. See also the thoughts of the eighteen-year-old Freud in an early letter on the "immoral in poetry" (Heinz Stanescu, *Unbekannte Briefe des jungen Sigmund Freud,* note 20, p. 128).
126. *Wiener Medizinische Wochenschrift,* 1887, col. 138. See also S. Freud, *G.W.,* Vol. 7 ("Civilized Ethics and Modern Nervous Illness"), pp. 143ff. In Hellpach's words (see note 119, p. 200): "The year 1880 marks the beginning of the insight into the disease of the nervous era"; words like "nervous," "nervousness," "hysteria," "neurasthenia" begin to become fashionable. See also Richard Hamann and Jost Hermand, "Epochen deutscher Kultur von 1870 bis zur Gegenwart" ("Epochs of German Culture from 1870 to the Present"), *Impressionismus,* Vol. 3, Munich, 1972, pp. 47ff.
127. Thus certain biographical circumstances in Freud's life might have been significant, e.g., his morally rigid life and, on the other hand, his exposure to sexual pathology in Charcot's patients years before. See note 94, pp. 431, 432.
128. *G.W.,* Vol. 16 ("A Disturbance of Memory on the Acropolis"), p. 250.
129. See note 8, p. 551. See also "Der Gehalt und die Funktion des Traumes im Werke Schnitzlers," in Gerd Klaus Schneider, *op. cit.,* pp. 232ff., and Reinhart Müller-Freienfels, *op. cit.,* pp. 31f.
130. *G.W.,* Vol. 2-3 (*The Interpretation of Dreams*), p. 101.
131. See note 8, p. 551.
132. See Gerhard Neumann and Jutta Müller, *op. cit.,* pp. 14, 157.
133. See note 4, p. 412.
134. See S. Freud, *Aus den Anfängen der Psychoanalyse. Briefe an Wilhelm Fliess. Abhandlungen und Notizen aus den Jahren 1887-1902* (*The Origins of Psycho-analysis: Letters to Wilhelm Fliess, Treatises and Notes from the years 1887-1902*), Frankfurt am Main, 1962, pp. 341ff.
135. See note 134, p. 345.

136. *G.W.,* Vol. 1 (*Studies on Hysteria*), p. 122.
137. See *G.W.,* Vol. 2-3 (*The Interpretation of Dreams*), pp. 110ff.
138. See note 65, p. 418. Heinz Politzer notes on Freud's *Interpretation of Dreams*s "Freud cherished a great love for dreams. He lets us understand how much he used to dream from early youth onward, unquietly and creatively, how much he was attached to his dreams. He offers them to his readers as if they were precious and fragile pieces in an archaeological cabinet." ("Freud als Deuter seiner Träume," p. 44.)
139. *G.W.,* Vol. 2-3 (*The Interpretation of Dreams*), p. 100.
140. *Ibid.,* p. 166.
141. See also Trudy Schmidt, "Bemerkungen zur Rezeption von Freuds *Traumdeutung*" ("Remarks on the Reception of Freud's *Interpretation of Dreams*"), *Psyche,* Vol. 26, 1972, pp. 707ff.
142. This throws light on William H. Reys's statement: "Without doubt the psychic researchers Schnitzler and Freud have much in common, but it would be false to assume that the characters of the creative writer were formed according to the prescription of the psychologist. Psychoanalysis thus does not deliver the key to understanding Schnitzler's work." See "Das Wagnis des Guten in Schnitzlers *Traumnovelle*" ("Risk of the Good in Schnitzler's *Traumnovelle*"), *The German Quarterly,* Vol. 35, 1962, p. 255). Completely apart from the fact that it is difficult to imagine that Schnitzler had drafted characters according to prescription, psychoanalysis doubtlessly does deliver keys (not the only ones) to the understanding of many a work as the treatise of Lotte S. Couch (see note 105) impressively shows. A diary note of Schnitzler's on September 17, 1912, likewise points in this direction. It notes a "stimulating conversation on dream interpretation and psychoanalysis" with Dr. Theodor Reik. He further notes "overestimation of the Oedipus complex by the Freudian school (to which Reik belongs). We analyzed Georg's dream together (*Weg ins Freie,* chapter 7)." The distance to Freud's *Interpretation of Dreams* may be shortened in the *Traumnovelle* as well, when one remembers that early sketches go back to 1907 and earlier. (See Hertha Krotkoff, *op. cit.,* note 85, p. 90.)
143. See note 21, p. 8.
144. How sensitively Freud makes his formulations may be seen in the fact that Josef Körner, who had published two longer works on Schnitzler before his death, wrote in one article of Schnitzler's "pessimism" and of the "erotic" which is "almost always experienced and represented oppressively." Schnitzler rejects these interpretations in extensive letters (see "Briefe an Josef Körner," *Literatur und Kritik,* Vol. 2, 1967, pp. 79ff.).
145. See note 1, p. 357.
146. See note 1, p. 104 ("Briefe an Arthur Schnitzler").

Feldbergstrasse 10
6500 Mainz
West Germany

FREUD'S LOVE LETTERS: Intimations of Psychoanalytic Theory

Ada Farber

During the four-year engagement of Sigmund Freud and Martha Bernays between the years 1882 and 1886, Freud wrote more than nine hundred letters to his fiancée.[8] Of these, Ernst Freud selected ninety-three for publication, not to illuminate the "theory and practice of psychoanalysis" but because he hoped that they would present a "portrait of the man" who wrote them.[1] Yet, regardless of the editor's intention, his father's correspondence is, in fact, rich in suggestions of the attitudes and ideas that Freud was later to develop into his theoretical structure.

The letters express the day-to-day concerns and struggles of a young doctor and his feelings about his fiancée as well as other people and events in his environment—his moods, aspirations, frustrations, successes, reversals, prejudices, and interests. Therefore, they provide us with an invaluable prism through which the ambience peculiar to the structure of bourgeois society in the late nineteenth century Vienna is refracted into its component values, attitudes, and customs. Social status and sex roles are but two aspects of the social environment that reveal themselves in the letters. It is the purpose of this essay to explore Freud's early thoughts in these two, often interlocking, areas, and to show how they are precursors of the concept of the superego in his fully developed theory. I suggest that there is a strong connection between the differences in the manner that men and women in *fin de siècle* Vienna were thought to acquire social status and the theory that the superego became, according to Freud's later thought, less completely formed in women than it did in men. It will become clear that these early, intimate expressions of the man who was to become the founder of psychoanalysis give us a

0033-2836/78/1300-0166 $00.95

special insight: we find in them not only something of the social context of his life, but also his particular, personal perspective within that context. My assumption is, of course, that this insight into Freud's social setting ought to deepen our understanding of his enormously complex and rich theory of personality, rather than to diminish it or explain it away.

The theory of psychoanalysis is well known, so there is no need to expatiate on it. The reader will be referred to appropriate sources for it so that I may give most attention to the content of the letters themselves and to their implications, explaining how they prefigure Freud's later concentration and elaboration.

The society of Freud's time made an extreme differentiation between the sexes, an emphasis which is evident from even a cursory glance at its costume, education, legal rights, and social roles. Freud himself made apparent in his letters to Martha that this was a matter of importance to him. Ultimately, he was to explain this difference in terms of the divergent manner the two sexes developed psychologically from infancy through the latency period—particularly as they encountered the castration and Oedipus complexes.[5a] Juliet Mitchell has done much to correct some widely held misapprehensions of Freud's ideas on masculinity and femininity.[7] In this important aspect of his theory he did not rule out social and cultural demands that were, in ways still unclear to him even in 1933, responsible for the particular qualities associated with femininity:

> We must beware . . . of underestimating the influence of social customs which force women into passive situations. All this is still far from being cleared up.[5b]

Yet, as early as 1883 he thought,

> A different education could suppress woman's delicate qualities—which are so much in need of protection and yet so powerful—with the result that they could make a living like men. [However,] all reforming activity, legislation and education, will founder on the fact that long before the age at which a profession can be established in our society, nature will have appointed woman by her beauty, charm, and goodness, to do something else. (*Letters,* p. 76)

This is from a letter attacking John Stuart Mill's essay, "The Enfranchisement of Women," which he had translated into German several years before while still a student. He clearly declared that the equality of women might be possible in some limited sense but was, in his view, a highly undesirable goal. Were it to come about, it would mean the "disappearance of the most lovely thing the world has to offer us: our ideal of Womanhood" (*Letters,* p. 76). Here we can see that the meaning of femininity was an important matter to Freud, that he was attached to the notion, prevalent in his time, of a feminine ideal, and perhaps most important, that he was intensely interested in sexual differentiation itself and its origins in nature or in custom.

What was this feminine ideal as we encounter it in the letters? First of all, there is a diachronic distinction to be drawn: the ideal has one characterization for a young woman, but a different one for an older woman.

> The position of woman cannot be other than what it is: to be an adored sweetheart in youth, and a beloved wife in maturity. (*Letters,* p. 76)

Then, as often happened in the correspondence, Freud fixed Martha in his scheme by the way he addressed her, writing a few lines later, "Farewell, my sweet girl." This passage is a positive statement of the ideal, and we will see below more precisely what it means. Further, so definite was the ideal that Freud elaborated it by employing the negative: women who did not conform to the ideal were often considered masculine (see below).

THE YOUNG PRINCESS

Freud's ideal young woman was attractive and aroused erotic romanticism in men while remaining passive herself. It was up to her suitor to draw her dependent affection away from her parents and to attach it to himself.

> And when you do return you are coming back to me, you understand, no matter how your filial feelings may rebel against it. From now on you are but a guest in your family, like a jewel that I have pawned and that I am going to redeem as soon as I am rich. For has it not been laid down since time immemorial that the woman shall leave father and mother and follow the man she has chosen?

> You must not take it too hard, Marty, you cannot fight against it; no matter how much they love you, I will not leave you to anyone, and no one deserves you; no one else's love compares with mine. (*Letters,* p. 23)

Although Martha's father had died when she was a little girl, Freud had his hands full in the task of taking Martha away from her mother, who, as we shall see, was a strong and determined woman in Freud's eyes. He pursued this end throughout the correspondence in a number of ways: in a stern, paternal manner he advised her against a relationship with her friend Elise (*Letters,* pp. 159-160); he counseled her on her reading, frequently referring to interesting and important literature that occupied him, especially if he found it suitable for a young woman in her early twenties (*Letters,* pp. 55, 88); often he expressed the wish, and occasionally he actually was able, to send her money for clothes of the latest fashion (*Letters,* p. 85); and when she was sick with a sore throat, greatly concerned he advised her, "to eat well, if necessary in secret, and if you need money for this, my sweet, just let me know" (*Letters,* p. 40). At this point Ernst Freud added a footnote explaining that the Bernays household adhered to the Jewish dietary laws. Apparently, Freud had scant confidence in Mama Bernays' chicken soup.

There were very many occasions on which Freud showed his opinion that Martha needed to be protected and that she was, and should be, dependent (*Letters,* pp. 162, 167, 186). His attitude is best summed up in the following passage:

> Just you wait, when I come you will soon get used to having a master again. And a severe one, too, but you couldn't have one who loves you more or who could be so deeply concerned about you. (*Letters,* p. 160)

While dependency was one attribute of the "young princess," as Freud frequently called her, erotic passivity was yet another. It seems to have been extremely important that the woman he fell in love with should not return his love immediately:

> I could never trust the love that responds to the first call and dismisses the right to grow and unfold with time and experience. (*Letters,* p. 153)

Clearly, Freud was speaking of Martha's response to his suit because a few lines later he added:

> From the moment I first saw you I was determined—no, I was compelled—to woo you, and how I persisted, despite all the warnings of common sense.

In other words, the ardor and intentions of the man were strong and spontaneous, very unlike those of his beloved, who was to be brought around by his slow, persuasive courtship:

> I really think I have always loved you much more than you me, or, more correctly, until we were separated you hadn't surmounted the *primum falsum* of our love—as a logician would call it—i.e., that I forced myself upon you and you accepted me without any great affection. I know it has finally changed and this success, which I wanted more than anything else, and the prolonged absence of which has been my greatest misery, gives me hope for the other successes which I still need. (*Letters,* p. 117)

It was not only in regard to his own engagement that Freud conveyed the idea that courtship consisted of masculine initiative overcoming girlish passivity. While describing relationships other than his own, he showed that the overcoming of feminine reticence was a pivotal aspect of the relations between the sexes and that it should be carried out by the man in the most gentle and delicate fashion. In a lengthy letter recounting the events leading to the suicide of a colleague, Nathan Weiss—a letter which reads like a story by Arthur Schnitzler—Freud attributed the tragedy to the character of the man:

> Weiss really was vitriol and he really did eat his way through everything. His gigantic self-importance was matched by an energy of an unusual kind, an ability to burrow his way into things and never let go. (*Letters,* p. 60)

These qualities brought Weiss success in many areas. But they were to bring about his downfall when applied to the sensitive associations with his bride. Against her will, he courted her until,

> At last she began to give in, thought she loved him, perhaps she had actually begun to feel some affection for him; she couldn't be

> certain. After all, no girl in love for the first time knows whether or not it is the real thing. (*Letters,* p. 63)

She was vacillating and undecided for a time and finally consented to the marriage, partly due to the pressure of her family:

> It is not difficult to guess why she had hesitated. I think he dropped his self-restraint too early, and physical aversion and moral disapproval quickly stifled all affection in the still cool and prudish girl. He on the other hand had believed that he could force love as he had forced all his other successes, and a false shame prevented him from letting the world know that he had been rejected. (*Letters,* p. 64)

Such a misapplication of masculine aggressiveness doomed the marriage at its inception, and a few weeks after it took place Weiss hanged himself.

That fascinating interpretation of sexuality makes this a very important letter. It is representative of the tone and quality of this aspect of the correspondence, and it illuminates, in part by negative example, his own feelings about his relationship with Martha. Even the salutations reflect his attitude. With one exception which will be discussed below, they are all diminutive endearments (see pp. 20-22). We observe his careful solicitude in general. It presents itself in the care with which he kept her up to date about his activities in minute detail, in the accounts of his feelings, and in the way he gradually introduced her to his sexual desire, which, in this collection, never went beyond kissing and embracing. One wonders whether this reticence is due to the fact that the editor is Freud's son, or whether the letters are, in this respect, representative.

On those occasions when he became carried away and did express anger with her or mentioned unpleasant subjects, he frequently followed such letters up, sometimes on the same day, with deep regret at his own lack of self-restraint, or at least he expressed the idea that their separation made it difficult to share the nuances of his feelings for her (*Letters,* pp. 161-162). At other times he was worried that she might idealize him and would be disappointed with him when, at last, they would be reunited (*Letters,* p. 89). Thus, he also feared the consequences of the very restraint that he felt to be so necessary.

In sum, Freud saw himself, and men generally, as aggressive and driving, while women were for him passive and innocent.

> I can hardly contain myself for silent savagery, and your latest letters are so tame; if you weren't such a sweet angel, I would love to have a good squabble with you. (*Letters,* p. 89)

The woman was conceived, in fact, to be so passive as to be unformed unless she became molded by the subtle hand of a masterful, self-controlled man. Whether this is an accurate self-appraisal is here not important.

Before leaving the subject of the young princess, I want to examine it in another aspect. In addition to Freud's very personal view, he was also extremely sensitive to the social implications of the mode of courtship of his time and to many of its ramifications in matters of status, such as wealth, profession, family, education, and reputation. The awareness of these implications imposed on him pressures of their own and provided some of the motivation for his feelings and behavior.

Wealth and Profession

For almost three and a half years of their engagement Martha lived in Wandsbek, a town outside of Hamburg, while Freud remained in Vienna. The unhappiness and privation brought about by this long separation clearly made Freud especially conscious of the conditions responsible for the delay in their marriage, chief among which were Freud's poverty and the smallness of Martha's dowry. These two factors, especially the former, were a frequent topic of the letters. Poverty came up in the very first letter[6] and subsequently was woven together with three other subjects.

The first of these was the inconveniences and irritations of everyday life: whether to eat in his room or go to cafes; debts of all kinds; the threadbareness of his clothes; the high prices of things; the question of whether to walk to make the house calls, or take a taxi.

The second subject was the effect of his poverty on Martha: how sorry she must feel for him (*Letters,* p. 49); how it prevented him from buying her presents (*Letters,* pp. 15, 45, 57, 58); how the expenses of a journey prevented them from seeing one another (*Letters,* p. 20); but, most important, how it delayed their marriage.

Because of their poverty their engagement and correspondence had, at first, to be in secret:

> . . . because as a poor man I should have to be ashamed of what everyone would reproach me with as injudicious thoughtlessness. Only Martha not, I hope.[6]

Freud revealed the social significance of money. It was, for both engaged partners, a social asset among others, and therefore, its possession made it possible for each to attract a mate with equal or higher social position:

> Woe to the day you become so rich that I, like a character in a bad novel, have to ask you politely whether you wish to continue to be my betrothed as I do not wish to stand in the way of your happiness. (*Letters,* p. 137)

Third, the question of money figured importantly also in determining the direction of Freud's career. Were he to continue his histological and neurological research at the University of Vienna he would have to wait for an indefinite time in order to become capable of supporting a wife. However, a career in the practice of medicine promised earlier financial independence but less prestige. Therefore, less than two months after he became engaged, he embarked on his work in the General Hospital in Vienna and applied himself to the formal study of the art of healing with the intention of setting up an independent practice as soon as possible.

He never felt completely at home in this and continued his interest in pure research:

> If you worry about having interfered with my scientific career I will laugh and tell you the story of Benedikt Stilling, a doctor who died a few years ago in Cassel, practiced science in his youth and was then compelled to take a job as a doctor. But for thirteen years he worked every morning on the human spinal cord, the result of which was a great work, and every evening he continued to work on the brain, and he is known as the foremost among the scientists to whom we owe the knowledge of this noble organ. (*Letters,* p. 71)

It is evident that the medical career was a compromise in order to provide them with a living, and was a difficult decision for Freud to make. The letters to Martha are full of accounts detailing conversations with established research scientists, Nothnagel, Meynert, Brücke, and Breuer, each of whom was instrumental in Freud's decision to continue making himself an independent practicing physician. These same men, because of their prestigious positions, were also important in helping him to climb the research ladder, which was the avenue to status in the medical field (*Letters,* pp. 30-34). His success as a scientist was an extremely important goal, and the details of the progress of his research, publications, and later on, his lectures, take up a large portion of the correspondence.

Youth

In addition to money, as well as "charm, beauty, and goodness" already mentioned in the letter about John Stuart Mill, a most important asset enabling a woman to attract a husband was her youth. Freud was extremely conscious of the fact that Martha would be growing older as their engagement dragged on, and he frequently expressed his appreciation of her willingness to wait:

> I had a talk today with a colleague in the hospital, Dr. Widder, who said he considers it a great mistake to marry as long as one has no money and that it will take me eight years to get anywhere. . . . Defending my case valiantly, I told him he just doesn't know my girl, who is willing to wait for me indefinitely, that I would marry her even if she had turned thirty—a matron. (*Letters,* p. 44)

> My girl must promise to keep young and fresh as long as possible, and even after nine years to be as charmingly surprised by everything new and beautiful as she is now. (*Letters,* p. 12)

> Courage, my treasure! You will become my wife much earlier and you won't have to feel ashamed of having had to wait so long. (*Letters,* p. 45)

> The poor sweet child [Martha], who has already suffered so many sad things which she doesn't mention, and hardly was she able to breathe again when she gave herself to the poor luckless man, renouncing so willingly her own little share of life's pleasure. (*Letters,* p. 28)

Much of the attractiveness that youth gave to a woman seemed to have consisted of the passive innocence already discussed, and to this innocence a woman's reputation, another vital asset, was closely linked. The extremely outraged reaction of Freud to Martha's association with her friend, Elise, in Wandsbek, attests to this. Freud felt that Martha's own reputation could be tarnished unless she desisted from being a "doormat" (*Letters*, p. 160) and abandoned plans the girls had for a visit:

> What is the good of your feeling that you are now so mature that this relationship can't do you any harm? A girl doesn't intentionally lower herself to irresponsible behavior such as your friend has always suggested and finally quite openly displayed. . . . Don't put yourself on the same level by keeping up friendly relations. (*Letters*, p. 160)

Freud was quite sensitive to the appeal of youthful femininity and to its usefulness in a social sense. This he made clear in casual observations about other girls as they appeared throughout the correspondence. In his account of Nathan Weiss, for example, he indicated that one of the reasons that the fiancée was willing to marry Weiss was the social pressure upon a woman who was still unmarried at the age of twenty-six. Speaking of his own sisters, he wrote condescendingly,

> By the way, Marty, little Pauli has already fallen happily in love, what do you think of that? With the 28-year-old brother of her girl friend, Glaser, with whom she used to spend her vacations. He has taken his law degree and is a junior counselor-at-law. . . . But doesn't it look as though our silly girls are very much in demand? Dolfi is the only one still unattached. (*Letters*, p. 108)

In a letter that recounts an important visit to Professor Nothnagel, Director of the Second Medical Clinic of Vienna, Freud wrote that he found himself waiting for the interview in a room on whose wall was a family portrait. Among the children was:

> A little girl with hints of potential beauty for whom within ten years the young men will be fighting at the students' balls. (*Letters*, p. 30)

Family

Still another dimension of status in which Freud displayed a keen interest was family position. He had the greatest respect for the reputation of Martha's grandfather, who had been a distinguished rabbi and the head of the Sephardic Community of Hamburg. Freud also wrote with admiration about Martha's two living uncles, both of whom had high-ranking university positions, a status to which Freud himself aspired. Michael Bernays was Professor of the History of Literature at the University of Munich, and Jacob Bernays was Professor of Classical Philology at Breslau and later at Bonn.

Freud's reverence for Martha's family background was most articulately expressed in a letter in which he described a fortuitous meeting he had with a Jew who had been a member of the congregation of Martha's grandfather. This old man extolled the accomplishments of the Bernays family (*Letters*, pp. 17-22). The decided pleasure and excitement that Freud had on this occasion is evident throughout the letter. Near its conclusion, he wrote:

> If my Marty wishes to take with her to Vienna some gifts in the form of notepaper [the old Jew had a shop where he sold it], she must go to the Adolphplatz, to our old Jew, disciple of her grandfather, and mention her name. Let him see that the stock of his master has not deteriorated since he sat at his master's feet. (*Letters*, p. 22)

Freud's own family was not so illustrious, and the "good stock" of Martha's ancestry seems to have made some contribution to his feelings for her.

There is a letter to Martha which I will quote at length because in it Freud himself summarized some of these attitudes about status and demonstrated how strongly he felt about them:

> Yesterday I went to see my friend, Ernst v. Fleishl, whom hitherto, so long as I did not know Marty, I envied in every respect. . . . He is a thoroughly excellent person in whom nature and education have combined to do their best. Wealthy, skilled in all games and sports, with the stamp of genius in his manly features, good-looking, refined, endowed with many talents and capable of forming an original judgment about most things, he has always been my ideal, and I was not satisfied until we became friends and I could properly enjoy his value and abilities. . . . Then I looked around his room, fell to thinking about my superior friend and it occurred to me how much he could do for a girl like Martha, what a setting he could provide for this jewel, how Martha, who was enchanted even by our humble Kahlenberg, would admire the Alps, the waterways of Venice, the splendor of St. Peter's in Rome; how she

> would enjoy sharing the importance and influence of this lover, how the nine years which this man has over me could mean as many unparalleled happy years of her life compared to the nine miserable years spent in hiding and near-helplessness that await her with me. I was compelled, painfully to visualize how easy it could be for him —who spends two months of each year in Munich and frequents the most exclusive society—to meet Martha at her uncle's [the Professor Michael Bernays] house. . . . Can't I too for once have something better than I deserve? Martha remains mine. (*Letters,* pp. 11-12)

In addition to the noble status of von Fleishl and his wealth, Freud had yet a more immediate reason to envy the man: von Fleishl had the professional standing that Freud wanted for himself. He was one of Brücke's assistants at the Physiological Institute where Freud was then a student doing research. Because there was no hope for advancement for many years there (Brücke was well satisfied with his two assistants), and because the situation was similar at the other research institutions, it had become evident to Freud that he should seek a position at the hospital clinic. Within the context of the complex of elements that comprised social status, we have arrived at a much fuller understanding of what Freud meant when he said that Martha was better than he "deserved."

THE HAUSFRAU

Since our sources are the love letters of Freud before his marriage, there is much less material in them to reveal how he thought of the woman in the role of wife. There are a few suggestions, though, to indicate that the wife had for him a noticeably different set of attributes. Once she was married, Freud expected a woman to be nurturing, orderly, devoted to her husband and children, and equal to her husband, but only within a very limited sphere of the household and in a peculiar sense.

The nurturing aspect is best illustrated by Freud's frequent description of the goodness and kindness of his future wife and of other wives of whom he approved. In the John Stuart Mill letter mentioned above, goodness was one of the distinctively feminine traits. Talking about the wife of a patient of his, Freud wrote:

> I admire her because she has excellent observation, nurses him with such patience and is so good at cheering him up. (*Letters,* p. 45)

The orderliness and dedication to her household that Freud anticipated in his future bride is vividly depicted in the following passages:

> Now it occurs to me that we would need two or three little rooms to love and eat in and to receive a guest, and a stove in which the fire for our meals never goes out. And just think of all the things that have got to go into the rooms! Tables and chairs, beds, mirrors, a clock to remind the happy couple of the passage of time, an armchair for an hour's pleasant daydreaming, carpets to help the housewife keep the floors clean, linen tied with pretty ribbons in the cupboard and dresses of the latest fashion and hats with artificial flowers, pictures on the wall, glasses for everyday and others for wine and festive occasions, plates and dishes, a small larder in case we are suddenly attacked by hunger or a guest, and an enormous bunch of keys—which must make a rattling noise. And there will be so much to enjoy, the books and the serving table and the cosy lamp, and everything must be kept in good order or else the housewife, who has divided her heart into little bits, one for each piece of furniture, will begin to fret. (*Letters,* p. 27)*
>
> I dare say we agree that housekeeping and the care and education of children claim the whole person and practically rule out any profession, even if simplified conditions relieve the woman of housekeeping, dusting, cleaning, cooking, etc. (*Letters,* p. 75)

The matter of equality is more difficult to pin down:

> I know after all how sweet you are, how you can turn a house into a paradise, how you will share in my interests, how gay yet painstaking you will be. I will let you rule the house as much as you wish, and you will reward me with your sweet love. (*Letters,* p. 71)

Freud, on several occasions, spoke of equality between Martha and himself as a goal, but he seems to have meant by this that they

---

* It is interesting to juxtapose this letter to a passage from Freud's account of his analysis of Dora:

> From the accounts given me by the girl [Dora] and her father I was led to imagine her [Dora's mother] as an uncultivated woman and above all as a foolish one, who had concentrated all her interests upon domestic affairs, especially since her husband's illness and the estrangement to which it led. She presented the picture, in fact, of what might be called the "housewife's psychosis." She had no understanding for her children's more active interests, and was occupied all day long in keeping them clean—to such an extent as to make it almost impossible to enjoy them. This condition, traces of which are to be found often enough in normal housewives, inevitably reminds one of forms of obsessional washing and other kinds of obsessional cleanliness.[3]

would have no secrets from one another, and that they should share their feelings about each other, even when these were unpleasant or disapproving (*Letters,* pp. 29-30). However, one has the impression that this is an equality of a very different kind than what the term calls to mind today. The equal status that Freud granted his future wife was one that she could accept only after she had been tamed and molded, a process that he was continually undertaking throughout the relationship in the correspondence. The fiancée was being transformed into the wife by her master. The result was to be a *hausfrau,* and a willing one, dedicated to her husband in the same way that Cordelia claimed herself to be to her future husband. This last was in a letter in which Freud told of a conversation with his esteemed colleague, Josef Breuer:

> And then I opened up and said [to Breuer]; "This same Martha . . . is in reality a sweet Cordelia. . . ." Whereupon he said he too always calls his wife by that name because she is incapable of displaying affection to others, even including her own father. And the ears of both Cordelias, the one thirty-seven and the other twenty-two, must have been ringing while we were thinking of them with serious tenderness. (*Letters,* p. 41)

Of the wife of a colleague in Paris:

> She is very quiet when the men are talking but takes an interest in everything, is kindness itself toward her husband who cannot do without a certain amount of selfish comfort, with the result that he is always saying to me, "There is only one Louise." She allows herself to be sent wherever he wants her to go, stays with him when he wants her to, looks after him and enjoys things with him. (*Letters,* p. 183)

There are some suggestions that the charm and erotic attractiveness of a woman were expected to recede in importance as an ideal attribute after she had become married, as, for instance, in the case of the above exemplary Louise who was "fat" and not at all attractive, but who had brought to her husband a substantial dowry in addition to having been from a good family and well educated (*Letters,* p. 183). I hesitate to make too much of this matter, since it is a point that is infrequently and subtly implied. At any rate, it can be said with some assurance that Freud felt that passivity in a woman should extend from courtship into marriage, that if she "ruled the household" she did so in so far as she had learned her place as devoted wife, and that if she had an independent intelligence or education, these resources were to be employed by her within the circumscribed setting of the home, with her husband as its supreme authority.

NEGATIVE ATTRIBUTES

The sharp dichotomy between the two sexes—that "humanity is divided between men and women, and that this difference is the important one" (*Letters,* pp. 75-76)—was an assumed condition, the elaboration of which was to become an important aspect of Freud's psychoanalytic theory. We have already seen the description of the girl and woman in positive terms. Yet Freud also made clear his feelings about what a woman ought not to be in a number of interesting passages. This negative femininity, when he detected it, was sometimes conceived of as a masculine quality and it was therefore considered to be undesirable in a female.

A most explicit statement of the negative woman appears in a letter about Martha's mother to Martha's sister, Minna, who was engaged to a close friend of Freud. In this letter Freud took it upon himself to advise Minna about the unsatisfactory turn that the relationship between Minna's fiancée and Mama Bernays had taken. Freud himself had an interest in this dispute because it concerned Mama's decision to move her household, along with her two daughters, from Vienna to Wandsbek:

> Now, I don't want you to think that I feel hostile to her [Mama] or that I have altered my high opinion of her or that I am on less affectionate terms with her. I do not think I am being unfair to her; I see her as a person of great mental and moral powers standing in our midst, capable of high accomplishments, without a trace of the absurd weaknesses of old women, but there is no denying that she is taking a line against us all, like an old man.* Because her charm and vitality have lasted so long, she still demands in return her full share of life—not the share of old age—and expects to be the center, the ruler, an end in herself. Every *man* [emphasis Freud's] who has grown honorably old wants the same, only in a

* At the time Martha's mother was fifty-three years old.

> woman one is not used to it. As mother she ought to be content to know that her three children are fairly happy, and she ought to sacrifice her wishes to their needs. This she doesn't do, she complains that she is superfluous and neglected, which we certainly give her no reason to feel; she wants to move to Hamburg at the behest of some extraordinary whim, oblivious of the fact that by so doing she would be separating you and Schönberg, Martha and myself for years to come. (*Letters,* p. 38)

In a number of passages that will follow Freud betrayed discomfort about aggressiveness, independence, or power in women, whereas he assumed these traits to be appropriate attributes in men. The interpretation that Elise's behavior mentioned above was demeaning, since she was a "poor girl who looks for a man" (*Letters,* p. 160), is an example of the transgression against the proper and customary right of the man to pursue the woman. In addition there are indications that he was ambivalent about Martha when she revealed these same strong feelings for him which he also sought to elicit from her:

> Don't consider me ungrateful or reproach me for thinking too little of you or seeming too cool. The more intimate your letters become, the more silent I get; as I read them something like a continual tacit assent goes on within me; yes, that is how I want my Marty to be, as she is now. (*Letters,* pp. 46-47)

In a most atypical letter in which Freud reproached Martha in a harsh, superior way for some unexplained (to us) behavior, it seems to be her independence from him that disturbed him especially:

> I acknowledge with pleasure the open admission of the cardinal baseness of your actions, for tradition has always interpreted a semiconfession on the part of a "lady" in this way, and even a beloved fiancée retains enough of the unassailable and unchangeable character of a "lady" for the man who loves her. You will allow me quietly to observe that you have been wrong on almost every point and without good reason, and have paid less attention to the whole business than you usually do to things concerning us both. Furthermore, you must allow me to point out that you could easily have changed everything according to your desire if only you had informed me about it. It is already quite some time now since I have been unyielding toward you, especially in small matters; a man will always get annoyed if his little woman appears to be try-

ing to get her own way by any other than straight means. If she is frank with him he will usually give in. (*Letters,* pp. 193-194)

In a jocular mood, he commented on the independence Martha displayed by traveling without the company of a man:

> My wandering princess
>
> Fancy, Lübeck! Should that be allowed? Two single girls travelling alone in North Germany! This is a revolt against the male prerogative, the beginning of the realization that one doesn't have to be lonely without a man. (*Letters,* p. 168)

Although the man was supposed to be in command, there are a number of letters indicating that Martha had some sort of power over Freud, a power often quite unsettling to him. He seems to have feared, at least somewhat, for instance, the extent to which his love for her affected his choice of profession. She sometimes left him confused, yet at other times she had what he thought was, and should be, a positive influence on his character. On the other hand, there were occasions when she made him lazy and lacking in ambition. Yet there are a few references to vague, inferior qualities of women. Following are several passages illustrating some of these ideas:

> To avoid arousing any suspicion I managed to be quite sociable. What sorceresses you women are! (*Letters,* p. 9)
>
> You are now even making me lazy, Marty. I do work all day, but in the evenings I am quite incapable of looking at a book. (*Letters,* p. 11)
>
> But you have got to bring me luck, for me you are luck itself, without you I would let my arms droop for sheer lack of desire to live; with you, for you, I will make use of them to gain our share in this world so as to enjoy it with you. (*Letters,* p. 28)
>
> Don't be cross my little girl, (whose charm at noon today is still confusing me). (*Letters,* p. 30)
>
> My dearest girl, if you dislike this kind of talk, just tell me to stop. You don't realize the extent of your influence over me and you must not conclude from the harsh way I deal with certain things connected with the basic conditions and experiences of our relationship that I am generally intolerant. I am quite prepared to be ruled by my princess. One willingly lets oneself be dominated by the person one loves; if only we had got as far as that, Marty! (*Letters,* p. 51)

> As my miserable person has taken on a greater importance, also for myself, since I acquired you, I am more concerned with my health and do not intend to wear myself out. I would rather renounce my ambition, attract less attention, have less success, than endanger my nervous system. In the future, for the remainder of my apprenticeship in the hospital, I think I shall try and live more like the Gentiles—modestly, learning and practicing the usual things and not striving after discoveries and delving too deep. My happiness lies above all in my relations with you, later in making you mine. (*Letters,* p. 54)

> What can it be that you want and do not dare to mention? . . . Something equally fantastic which would mean putting on my armor at once and setting out for the Orient? . . .
>
> Or is my sweetheart's desire nearer home; could it possibly be a deed of self-conquest? Am I to fast at Yom Kippur or reconcile myself to someone I don't like? Surely not. My Marty would not abuse her power and persuade me to actions that lack sense as well as honesty. I hope she wants something for herself and I hope I can catch it and give it to her. (*Letters,* p. 55)

> Continually having so much to do acts as a kind of narcotic. . . . Strange creatures are billeted in my brain. . . . The whole of medicine is becoming familiar and fluid to me. . . . When a letter from you arrives, the whole dream fades, life enters my cell. Then all the strange problems creep away, the mysterious pictures of diseases fade, and gone are the empty theories "according to the present status of the science," as they are invariably called. (*Letters,* p. 68)

> And you will reward me with your sweet love by rising above all those weaknesses for which women are so often despised. (*Letters,* p. 71)

Nowhere in the correspondence did Freud seem as inconsistent and ambivalent toward her as when he was struck by her power to "dominate" him, for good or evil, when he perceived her other than passive and dependent. What is more, the presence of an independent intelligence in a woman made him reveal his attraction as well as his fear:

> Marty, does it annoy you to hear me talk about such things? Oh, you won't be annoyed, you are so good and—between ourselves—you write so intelligently and to the point that I am just a little afraid of you. I think it all goes to show once more how quickly women outdistance men. Well, I am not going to lose anything by it. (*Letters,* p. 67)

It is noteworthy that the only letter that begins by addressing Martha by her name rather than by the nickname Marty or by a diminutive endearment—the only letter, among the ones published, which begins with "My beloved Martha"—is one in which he was commenting upon and responding to some "intelligent" discussion she had written about behavior of the "masses" at the Wandsbek Fair. He even compared her thinking to that of "Wagner in *Faust*" (*Letters,* p. 50). In this acknowledgment of her intellect, I think we must recognize a rare acceptance of some kind of true equality in his fiancée as a thinking, independent person.

I believe that this ambivalence underlies Freud's later theory of the development of the female personality. At least it may be said that the disturbing divergence between the prevalent passive, dependent ideal to which he was dedicated and his awareness, nevertheless, that women did have aggressive and independent drives in a sense cried out for an explanation. And it was the effort to arrive at this explanation that later occupied him.

THE MAN

While my discussion until this point has had women as its primary focus, it has, of necessity, included much about Freud's conceptions of men. Let me now direct attention onto men themselves.

A most prominent feature of the correspondence is the persistent picture one gets of Freud and the men with whom he worked and dealt as ambitious and driving. They were almost always presented in terms of the degrees to which their ambitions were realized—in terms of their success or failure. Achievements were acknowledged only in a limited number of areas: professional recognition in research and its publication; wealth; social position in a status hierarchy.

Freud was extremely preoccupied with his career. A very large and frequent theme of the correspondence was his progress, often in the minutest details, of the vicissitudes of his researches. He was nearly always working on a project or on its publication, and was explicitly concerned with the degree to which he was recognized for his achievements:

> Then I went to Breuer, whom I found rather cantankerous after his luncheon: his microscope was not quite in order. As a result I

wasn't able to show him everything, but what he did see drew from him quite a number of admiring comments. Then he said: "Now that you have the weapon, I wish you a happy war." No doubt it will mean a great deal of work before the first paper can appear, of which my little woman will receive an offprint. The great question is: Will this method also be suitable for tracing the fine nerve fibers in the tissues, in the skin, in the glands, etc. (*Letters,* p. 73)

Apart from its practical importance, this discovery has an emotional significance as well. I have succeeded in doing something I have been trying to do over and over again for many years. When I survey the time since I first began to tackle this problem, I realize that my life has progressed. . . . The same men whom I have admired from afar as inaccessible, I now meet on equal terms and they show me their friendship. (*Letters,* p. 73)

For a week now there has been a foreigner in the Salpêtrière, a definitely Germanic type and yet somehow different; I can't quite make him out. Wednesday is the day we go to the opthalmological room, and there this foreigner suddenly began behaving with some authority; when he exchanged cards with Charcot's opthalmologist, the latter became very polite and expressed the hope that Monsieur would often return so that he could learn something from him. Whereupon we all began wondering who he might be. Before leaving he came over to us Viennese and said: "I heard you speaking German. I'd like to introduce myself." My *bête noire* [a colleague whom Freud held in contempt] exchanged cards with him first and I was still trying to find mine when the foreigner said. . . . "Could you be Dr. F. from Vienna? I've known your name for a long time, from your publications, especially the one on cocaine." I was a little surprised and enquired after his name, which turned out to be Knapp. Now Knapp is the foremost opthamologist in New York. . . . I greeted him accordingly and my *bête noire* stood there looking rather sheepish. . . . When he heard the word cocaine mentioned he asked: "Have you also written on cocaine?" Whereupon Knapp replied: "Of course he has, it was he who started it all." This morning my Viennese [the *bête noire*] was much more malleable and talked exclusively of the great practice that awaited me in Vienna. (*Letters,* pp. 208-209)

Perhaps the discussion on courtship above gives sufficient evidence of Freud's consciousness of wealth. In addition, he had a great sensitivity to other symbols of social status and was made most keenly aware of them during his stay at the Salpêtrière of Charcot in Paris. Aside from the struggle for professional recognition in which he engaged there, he detailed for Martha a few social events at the Charcot residence, where he felt that he was entering a social circle above the ones to which he was accustomed and to which he felt he belonged.

Freud saw his social position as above the common masses who were without ambition because they were helpless and destined to poverty:

> When I see the people indulging themselves, disregarding all sense of moderation, I invariably think that this is their compensation for being a helpless target for all the taxes, epidemics, sicknesses, and evils of social institutions. (*Letters*, p. 51)

Above the masses were a middle and upper class in which men strove to make headway. In these letters one finds a chronicle of Freud's struggle to raise his social position from what appears to have been a solid, respectable, but poor middle class beginning. His engagement to a woman whose family occupied a higher class position—a position of which he was extremely conscious—might be considered to be an aspect of that struggle. However, the professional circle with its exacting demands of scientific work, its opportunities to make careful use of personal contacts to further one's ends, and its emblem of publication, was his main competitive arena.* It must by now be clear that for the young Freud women were not participants in this professional competition.

CONCLUSION

There are two general elements in Freud's social environment that can be distilled from the letters as I have reviewed them. Both deal with sexuality and both, more or less explicitly, have been incorporated into the theory of the Oedipus complex and how it is differentially encountered and resolved by the two sexes.

The first element is the presence of severe distinctions between the sexes in the ideal. Women were expected to be extremely dependent and passive and men extremely aggressive. Yet, even in this early period, Freud was also quite aware of the fact that the reality often departed from the ideal: that there were, in fact, women who had masculine qualities, or that even "feminine" women betrayed "masculine" traits. This would imply that a purely anatomical ex-

* Another area where Freud conveyed his concern about status lay in the connection he seems to have made between being a Jew and being ambitious (*Letters*, pp. 54, 71).

planation of sexuality would not be satisfactory. He was later to state "that what constitutes masculinity or femininity is an unknown characteristic which anatomy cannot lay hold of."[5c]

It should be stressed that the extreme differentiation of sex roles, and the fact that this differentiation was made so much of, were to have an influence upon Freud's questioning of the principle of anatomical determinism. Such an elaborate social ideal of femininity must have made transgressions and exceptions frequent and apparent, even prominent. In this social setting, any theory that explains the sexes would have to mediate between the cultural imperative of elaborate and extreme ideal differences on the one hand, and the egregious exceptions that such an imperative brought into focus on the other. That is precisely what Freud's developmental theory of sexual personality accomplishes:

> Psychoanalysis does not try to describe what a woman is—that would be a task it could scarcely perform—but sets about enquiring how she comes into being, how a woman develops out of a child with a bisexual disposition.[5b]

In other words, a paradoxical conclusion one comes to after reading these published letters is that Freud became sensitized to the similarity between the sexes—to human bisexuality—very much within the setting that demanded exaggerated sex role distinctions.

The second element of the social environment is related to the first. It is an aspect of sex role differentiation and involves, specifically, how a member of each sex was expected to perform his or her role. In precisely what sense was the man thought of as aggressive and active by Freud in the letters? Almost entirely in matters of status. Very few of the letters contain no mention of some effort on the writer's part to enhance his status, whether in the realm of "deserving" Martha, or making contacts to attain the position in a hospital or a research institute, or in descriptions of arduous, time-consuming and exhausting work that would lead to recognition through publication or reputation. This, in fact, was the active, aggressive, ideal man.

I find in the letters a series of privations that can only be described in terms of deferred gratification, and this is linked with masculine self-restraint, goal consciousness, and initiative. Without his explicitly saying so anywhere, so far as I know, striving for status goals with all that it entails is what Freud, at least in part, seems to mean in his developed theory by the transformation of aggression in the formation of the superego in men. The boy, as the result of his fear of castration brought about by his Oedipal longing for his mother, represses his hostile aggression against his father. This repressed, internalized aggression develops into the superego. The two parts of the superego in his theoretical structure, the conscience and the ego-ideal,[4] coincide with aspects of Freud's own adjustment to the social setting as I found it represented in the letters: (1) a complex and vivid ego-ideal in the form of professional and social goals; (2) a powerful conscience that imposed restraints on his relationship with Martha and that kept him doggedly working even in spite of enormous difficulties, privations, and tendencies to what he called laziness.

In contradistinction to the man who is active and aggressive in enhancing his status in the letters, and who has a fully developed superego in the theory, is the woman. From the letters one has the impression that she had no active means to attain higher status except by enhancing the gifts that family or nature had granted her. Thus, she was to use what "beauty, youth, charm" (and other assets mentioned earlier) she had and make the most of them. Is this not incorporated into the concept, in Freud's theory, of female narcissism in which a passive aim is actively sought? "Thus we attribute a larger amount of narcissism to femininity, which also affects women's choice of object, so that to be loved is a stronger need for them than to love."[5d] It was, in fact, by means of putting her vanity to use that a woman could attract a suitor, according to the ideal projected in the letters, and this method was one of her most important means for improving her social status.

Parallel to this "passive" way of coping with status (in the letters) is the stunted superego of the woman in the Freudian theoretical structure. Unlike the boy, the girl does not fear castration because she is already without a penis.

> The castration complex prepares for the Oedipus complex instead of destroying it; the girl is driven out of her attachment to her mother through the influence of her envy for the penis and she enters the Oedipus situation as though into a haven of refuge. In the absence of fear of castration the chief motive is lacking which leads boys to surmount the Oedipus complex. Girls remain in it for an in-

determinate length of time; they demolish it late, and even so, incompletely.[5e]

Freud created the concept of the superego as a mechanism whereby instinct was transfigured and gratification was postponed. The social structure, with its strong and intricate status orientation, was the setting for the development of the the theory in which Freud saw instinctual energy continually channeled into a powerful dual process, the prod of anticipated satisfaction (including romantic union) promised by the future attainment of the ego-ideal, and the restraint imposed by conscience. By means of this carrot and stick device, civilized humans were doomed to an existence in which their instinctual tensions were, at best, only partially released.* Important for the thesis of this essay is the notion that a significant aspect of the process was the implicit promise of fulfillment by means of the attainment of higher social status and recognition. Freud seemed at the time of the letters not to question the promise of fulfillment, but as his theories matured, he grew more and more pessimistic about the possibility of human happiness and satisfaction, so that the postponement of gratification, though necessary, made future happiness not much more than an illusion.

* This is most poignantly expressed by Freud in *Civilization and Its Discontents.*[2]

REFERENCES

1. Freud, Ernst L. (Ed.). *Letters of Sigmund Freud.* New York: Basic Books, 1961, p. viii. Henceforth this book will be cited in the text as *Letters.*
2. Freud, Sigmund. *Civilization and Its Discontents.* New York: Norton, 1962.
3. ———. *Dora: An Analysis of a Case of Hysteria.* New York: Collier, 1963, pp. 34-35.
4. ———. *The Ego and the Id.* New York: Norton, 1962, pp. 18-29.
5. ———. *New Introductory Lectures on Psychoanalysis.* New York: Norton, 1964, pp. (a) 112-135; (b) 116; (c) 114; (d) 132; (e) 129.
6. Jones, Ernest. *The Life and Work of Sigmund Freud.* New York: Basic Books, Vol. I, 1953, p. 105.
7. Mitchell, Juliet. *Psychoanalysis and Feminism.* New York: Pantheon, 1974, pp. 113-119.
8. Roazan, Paul. *Freud and His Followers.* New York: Knopf, 1975, p. 47.

1415 Hillcrest Road
Lancaster, Pennsylvania 17603

BOOK REVIEW

MINUTES OF THE VIENNA PSYCHOANALYTIC SOCIETY VOL. 3. Herman Nunberg and Ernst Federn (Eds.). New York: International Universtities Press, Inc., 1974. xviii + 367 pp.

Volume 3 includes weekly minutes of the Society and covers the period October 5, 1910, through December 20, 1911. The intellectual atmosphere of these meetings was rather plodding, as the discussants reached for additional areas that could be explained by the correlated concepts of libido and unconscious process. Notable exceptions were presentations by Adler and Stekel, which retain the intellectual ferment of the earlier years of the psychoanalytic movement. The years 1910 and 1911 were a time of transition in which Freud's first instinct theory was rapidly outgrowing its usefulness while the inevitable next step, toward a theory of aggression, had not yet been formulated. In this climate both Adler and Stekel presented theories stressing an aggressive drive, Adler focusing more on the drive for mastery and power, Stekel portraying aggression as a destructive "criminal" drive. Freud and his other followers in the Vienna Society (Sadger, Rank, Federn, Tausk, and Sachs, to name a few) were still busily unearthing offshoots of libido and viewing libido as the source of both health and neurosis, while viewing aggression as a side issue. Adler especially, and Stekel too, soon became nuisances by pushing aggression into the foreground as the source of health and neurosis, while tending to relegate libido to a side issue. The resulting atmosphere was potentially explosive, because Freud viewed both of them with suspicion, as detractors of his view. The outcome was inevitable. First Adler (during 1911) and then Stekel (a year or so later) were not so gently squeezed out of the Society as though they were psychoanalytic antichrists.

Psychoanalysis was dealt a severe blow by these acts of intolerance and narrow-mindedness, which were to serve as a warning to future detractors and set the scene for intolerance to new ideas, something which still plagues the psychoanalytic movement. This turmoil within the Society during 1910 and 1911 stands out more than the subject matter of the ongoing discussions.

0033-2836/78/1300-0190 $00.95 © 1978 N.P.A.P.

The discussants reached into many other fields for their subject matter: the choice of a profession, mother love, magic, poetry, writers, handwriting. Topics closer to the clinical mainstream included hysterical lying, the two principles of mental functioning, guilt, dreams, body erotism, masochism, and masturbation. Considering that the weekly meetings included original papers, many of which were subsequently published, the Society appears remarkable for its prodigious output, even though many presentations were crude and prosaic.

Through all the meetings Freud stands out as the personal and intellectual leader, as well as the undisputed boss. Freud was building an intellectual movement in which he personally trained and steered his disciples to add to the views he himself presented. Freud's evenness of temperament seems remarkable in view of the constant irritation caused by Adler and Stekel. It is questionable whether Freud should have been irritated but, since he was, his gentlemanly behavior was much to his credit. His irritation as leader and trend-setter was unfortunate, since in Adler's theories lay the beginnings both of a new instinct theory in which aggression would be the equal of libido, and of an ego psychology. Adler was able to see through the untenable concept of ego libido and view the ego as the seat and the instrument of aggression, a view Freud took only in part and at a later date. Freud could not tolerate Adler's rebellion, considering it destructive to psychoanalytic theory.

Adler emerges as an impetuous, sometimes impertinent, and occasionally even obnoxious, presence, but he is brilliant and stimulating throughout and the most interesting single driving force in the Society other than Freud himself. But Freud's earlier conflict with the genius of Breuer was repeated in new bad feelings toward Adler and other potentially giant presences of differing persuasion. Adler never had a chance. The battle between Adler and Freud was waged around working premises on Freud's side and around new perspectives and daring intellectual thrusts on Adler's side. Over and over again the group, following Freud's example, chastised Adler for being one-sided and for elevating secondary embellishments on human character into primary explanatory positions. Adler was accused, as had been Breuer twenty years earlier, of neglecting the importance of sexuality as the prime force in life. Additionally, he was accused of foresaking the concept of the unconscious in favor of a psychology of consciousness. Aided by Stekel's insistence on a criminal drive, one up even on Adler's concept of a power drive, Freud and most of his followers in the Society first made it impossible for Adler to remain and save face, and then began the attack on Stekel as well.

Originality in psychoanalysis has never been popular, except on approved home grounds, as a back-up force for the already acceptable. In 1910 and 1911 it was not simply Adler's future that was at stake. It was psychoanalysis itself, as the bastion of potential intellectual ferme In his lifetime Freud singlehandedly pushed for new explorations to promote his creation, psychoanalysis. With the passing of Freud lesser leaders emerged who needed all the help they could get. Freud could do without an Adler, but we cannot. And yet, even now the restrictiveness of what is acceptable has created a system of multiple leaders with mutual intolerance and, thus, with contributions often of dubious value. The Adler affair set a trend in dealing with dissidents. What remains are pockets of narcissism with accompanying clusters of followers, each cluster being suspicious of the others, each vying to replace Freud as supreme arbiter of the intellectually acceptable.

The years 1910 and 1911 were overly personal, not vintage, years for psychoanalysis, and there have been few vintage years since. *The Minutes of the Vienna Psychoanalytic Society* attests to the drive for conformity which even great men foster as soon as greatness becomes tarnished by the need to sustain and increase personal power. The editors are to be thanked for making available this careful and unbiased rendering of the minutes.

Irving Shuren